Keto Diet for Women Over 50

How to Lose Weight Eating Healthy and Tasty Food at 50 and Over

Maya Bryce

2

3

Table of Contents

Introduction

The ketogenic diet, or "keto" for short, is a way of eating that reduces your intake of carbohydrates such as bread, pasta, soda, starchy vegetables, sugar, and sweets, while increasing your fat consumption. Following a keto diet can be beneficial to your health and help you meet your weight loss goals. It can also improve, and in some cases reverse, many health conditions such as type 2 diabetes, heart disease, epilepsy, cancer, and Alzheimer's disease.

Your body burns sugars, which are found in carbohydrates, and fats throughout the day to give you energy. When you reduce your intake of carbohydrates, your body is no longer able to use these sugars as an energy source and switches to burning fat instead. This process is called ketosis, and it forms the foundation of the keto diet.

When your body is in ketosis and it has burned through the fats you have eaten throughout the day, it will begin to further target your stored fat, and, as a result you will find that your metabolism has improved, and you will start to lose weight.

With the health benefits plus the possibility of losing weight while still eating all of your favorite foods, it is no wonder that the keto diet has become exceedingly popular worldwide, especially among celebrities like Halle Berry, the Kardashians, and LeBron James.

Due to the increase in popularity, there are several different versions of the keto diet that have come about, including:

- **The standard keto diet** is the original keto diet that most people follow and the one that we will be focusing on in this book. This version of the keto diet reduces your intake of carbohydrates to 50 grams or less, while being high in fat and including moderate amounts of protein.

- **The targeted keto diet** is a version of the keto diet that is mostly used by athletes and people who are active in sports and weight training. This version of the keto diet is similar to the standard keto diet but before or after a workout session includes an additional 20-30 grams of carbohydrates to give your body that extra energy it needs to push itself harder and perform more intense workouts. If you are training or exercising, you should not pick up additional weight from consuming extra carbohydrates because they will likely be burned off during your workout session. However, if you are not training or you do not feel you need an extra boost during your workout sessions, I would suggest that you follow the standard keto diet instead.

- **The high-protein keto diet** reduces your intake of carbohydrates while including more protein and slightly less fat than the standard keto diet. With this version of the keto diet, your body will not go into ketosis, but you will still be able to lose weight and receive health benefits like you would with the standard keto diet. Your body can use the glucose that is converted from the protein as an alternative energy source.

- **The cyclical keto diet** is also a version of the keto diet that is mostly used by athletes and people who are active. The cyclical keto diet follows the same principles as the standard keto diet for five days of the week, followed by two days that are high in carbohydrates. Some people use this method on special occasions, such as a birthday or a wedding, when they know that they will be unable to stick to their diet. As the name suggests, your body will cycle in and out of ketosis. However, I suggest that you do not do this often, especially if you are following the diet for weight loss, as you will not lose as much weight with this version of the diet when compared to the standard keto diet.

The keto diet is often compared to similar diets like the Atkins diet and banting. Keto, the Atkins diet, and banting are all diets that are low in carbohydrates and high in fats with moderate amounts of protein.

The difference between keto and Atkins is that the Atkins diet is more complex, comprising four phases as you proceed through the diet. In phase one, you start out with 20-25 grams of carbohydrates per day and gradually increase your intake of carbohydrates as you continue to phase two through four. Phase four is the maintenance phase, and you will consume 80-100 grams of carbohydrates each day, which is more than with the keto diet.

Meanwhile, the difference between keto and banting is that keto is a more structured diet, while banting is less strict. Banting is more focused on including more meats, fruits, and vegetables into your diet, while the standard keto diet does not have as much emphasis on consuming as much protein and focuses instead on a high fat intake. There are also multiple phases in the banting diet, like with the Atkins diet.

The keto diet is recommended above all other similar diets to ensure that you meet your maximum health and weight loss goals.

Chapter 1: Your Body at 50

Turning 50 is a big milestone in your life, and it brings about many changes, both in your family life and to your body physically. Maybe your children have left the house to go to college or to settle down and start their own family, and you find that you have more time on your hands than you know what to do with. Or maybe you have noticed that your hair is turning grey at a faster rate, that your eyesight and hearing are no longer what they used to be, and that you have aches and pains that you never had before.

Turning 50 is different for everyone. You might be excited to start a new adventure, or you are not prepared at all and are dreading the changes that are coming. But no matter what your take on turning 50 is, you cannot stop it from happening. So, now is the time to take control of your life, eat healthy food, lose weight, and prepare your body for the next stage of your life so that you can face everything that comes your way with confidence and grace.

Here are some of the changes you will be experiencing as you turn 50 or over:

- **Your metabolism slows down.** Even before you turn 50, you might have noticed that your metabolism has started to slow down. However, at 50 and over, this becomes more noticeable than before. You might find that you are gaining weight from eating the same foods that you ate when you were younger to maintain your weight. What this means is that as you get older and your metabolism slows down, you

18

should eat smaller food portions if you want to maintain the same weight that you did before and eat significantly less than that if you want to lose weight.

- **Your bones become brittle.** When your body goes through menopause and your estrogen levels decrease, the rate at which your bones deteriorate increases, making your bones become more brittle. It is important that you begin strength training to keep you strong and prevent further bone loss, which could result in injuries.
- **Your muscles will become weaker.** The rate at which you lose muscle mass is another factor that is affected by menopause when hormones like estrogen are reduced in your body. When you experience muscle loss, your muscles will become weaker. I suggest that

you include endurance training, such as lifting weights and high-intensity interval training, to continue to strengthen your muscles.

- **You may experience problems with your digestive system.** As you go through menopause and postmenopause, your body and hormones will change. When your metabolism slows down and your muscles become weaker, your stomach muscles will struggle to digest some foods, such as dairy and gluten. As a result, you will experience problems with your digestive system like bloating or constipation. If you are experiencing digestive issues, you should cut out foods one at a time to see which one is giving your stomach problems. Once you have identified the culprit, you can either try and avoid eating it, if for example you have become lactose intolerant, or eat the problem food in smaller amounts so that you can reduce your chances of developing digestion problems.

- **You will struggle to lose weight.** When you get older and your metabolism slows down, you will notice that you are unable to lose weight as effectively as you used to. This is because as we get older our bodies struggle to convert fat into energy that can then be used throughout the day, especially when you are including other energy sources in your diet like carbs. As a result, your body will retain the fat that you consume, and you will struggle to lose it.

- **You may develop arthritis.** If you have someone in your family that is suffering from arthritis, then there is an increased chance that you will develop it in your 50s or older. By staying active and exercising, you could decrease your symptoms and reduce any inflammation and pain that you may experience. By keeping your body moving, you could reduce the risk of having an arthritis attack.

- **Your body will struggle to produce protein.** As you get older, you will need to consume more protein because your body will no longer be as effective at producing and retaining protein. When you are not including enough protein in your diet, you can experience muscle loss and weakness. By including more protein in your diet, you will be able to maintain your muscle mass for longer.

- **Your brain function may weaken.** If you do not continuously learn new things and exercise your brain, your brain function could deteriorate. When your brain function weakens, you could have trouble remembering things or develop memory loss, and your attention span could decrease. You can continue to exercise your brain and develop your brain function by breaking your daily routine and doing something out of the ordinary, meeting new people, and experiencing new events and locations.

What Nutrients Does My Body Need at 50?

Once you are aware of the changes that you might experience at 50 and over, you should find out more about what nutrients your body needs and be sure to include them in your diet. Below I have listed some of the main nutrients that will be beneficial to your diet as you get older.

Protein

Protein is an important nutrient that your body needs to provide structure and maintenance to your cells and tissues and acts as a source of energy that your body can use to fuel itself throughout the day.

Protein is also used by your body to maintain muscle mass and reduce muscle loss, improve your immune system to fight off bacteria and infections, and produce enzymes which cause metabolic reactions in your body, such as digestion.

Protein can be found in animal products such as beef, chicken, eggs, fish, and tuna, as well as in almonds, broccoli, brussels sprouts, and dairy products like cottage cheese and plain Greek yogurt.

To calculate how much protein you should be consuming every day, you should first weigh yourself. For every kilogram of your body weight, it is recommended that you have a protein intake of 0.8 grams. Therefore, if you weigh 70 kilograms, then you should include 56 grams of protein per day in your diet.

Calcium

Calcium is another essential nutrient that you need in your diet that your body cannot produce on its own. It is especially important as you get older and experience bone loss. Calcium helps with a number of functions in your body, such as strengthening your teeth and bones and circulating blood and nutrients around your body.

You can find the best sources of calcium in dairy products such as cheese and plain Greek yogurt. However, if you are lactose intolerant or vegan, you will need to look at other sources of calcium, for example, calcium-fortified foods. Almonds, sardines, figs, and leafy greens like broccoli, kale, and spinach contain good sources of calcium, and you can include these in your diet.

For our bodies to absorb calcium, you will also need to ensure that you are including enough vitamin D in your diet. You can get vitamin D from foods like salmon, sardines, egg yolks, mushrooms, and fortified foods that have vitamin D added to them. Sunlight also provides you with a natural source of vitamin D.

A woman at the age of 50 should take 1,000 mg of calcium and 600 IU of vitamin D in their diet every day. Meanwhile, women over the age of 51 should increase their calcium intake to 1,200 mg, and women over the age of 70 should increase their daily vitamin D intake. You can take a calcium supplement if you are struggling to include the recommended amount in your diet.

Fiber

Fiber is a nutrient that helps to improve your metabolism, digest the food that you eat, keep your bowel movements regular, and lose weight, and keeps your blood sugar levels steady. Fiber can be a beneficial nutrient to consume in your diet and can assist in improving health conditions like diabetes.

Foods that are sources of fiber include all leafy greens, such as broccoli, brussels sprouts, and lettuce, as well as avocado, tomato, some berries, nuts like almonds and walnuts, and seeds like chia, flax, and hemp.

It is recommended that you include 25 grams of fiber every day in your diet. I suggest that you include a fiber supplement for the first few days if you are changing your diet to help you remain regular as your body gets used to the new foods.

Vitamin B12

Vitamin B12 is an essential nutrient that you should include in your diet. It helps to strengthen your brain function and keeps it from deteriorating as you get older, and it helps to produce oxygenated red blood cells that are transported through your body.

Vitamin B12 is found in animal products such as dairy, beef, chicken, eggs, and fish. If you are a vegetarian or vegan, vitamin B12 will be harder to include into your diet, but there are some fortified food alternatives, such as dairy, that you can use that have vitamin B12 added.

After 50, you have a greater risk of developing a vitamin B12 deficiency, which can be dangerous to your health. If there is concern that you are not receiving enough vitamin B12 in your diet, it is recommended that you consider taking a vitamin B12 supplement and including fortified food alternatives in your diet.

It is recommended that if you are over the age of 50 you should take 500 mcg of vitamin B12 each day and up to 1,000 mcg in more severe cases of deficiency.

Potassium

Potassium is a nutrient that you should include in your diet that helps your body to function properly by helping to improve digestion, stabilize your blood pressure, improve the signals that are transmitted along nerves in your body, and reduce your risk of osteoporosis and stroke. You can also use potassium as an electrolyte to replenish lost fluids in your body.

Foods that are sources of potassium include avocado, mushrooms, meat, salmon, almonds, hemp seeds, and leafy greens, such as broccoli, brussels sprouts, and spinach.

There is no specific amount of potassium that you are required to include in your diet, but it is suggested that you have 3,500 mg each day to ensure that you don't develop a deficiency. You can include a potassium supplement if you are not consuming enough potassium in your diet.

Magnesium

Magnesium is another nutrient that you should include in your diet to ensure proper bodily functions. Magnesium helps with DNA synthesis, improves the signals that travel from your nerves to your brain, and stabilizes your blood pressure and blood sugar levels.

Foods that are sources of magnesium include almonds, avocados, spinach, and tofu.

It is recommended that a woman over the age of 50 should have 320 mg of magnesium each day. You can also include a magnesium supplement into your diet if you have a magnesium deficiency. One of the signs of a magnesium deficiency that I have noticed is that you might experience muscle cramps. By taking a magnesium supplement, you can reduce this occurrence.

Iron

Iron is an essential nutrient that your body needs so that oxygenated blood can be transported around your body.

Foods that are sources of iron include broccoli, spinach, tuna, shellfish, red meat, turkey, organ meats such as liver, kidneys, brain, and heart, as well as tofu and pumpkin seeds.

The amount of iron that you should have each day depends on various factors, such as your age, diet, genetics, and whether you are still menstruating or not. A woman who is 50 years old should take 18 mg of iron each day. However, if you are 51 and older, you will decrease your intake to 7 mg each day.

Even if you do not have an iron deficiency, I would recommend that you get an iron supplement. You can take it if you feel like you have no energy for the day or if you haven't gone through menopause yet and are nearing your cycle.

Omega-3 Fats

Omega-3 fats are an essential nutrient that your body needs to help maintain and protect brain function and eyesight, and to improve your immune system against illnesses such as ADHD, breast cancer, and depression, as well as inflammatory diseases like arthritis.

Foods that contain omega-3 fats include anchovies, chia seeds, cod liver oil, flax seeds, herring, mackerel, oysters, salmon, sardines, and walnuts.

If you are including fatty fish in your diet at least two times a week, then you should be meeting your omega-3 dietary requirements. However, if you are not receiving enough omega-3 in your diet, then it is recommended that you take an omega-3 supplement.

Nutrients You Should Avoid at 50

Trans Fats

Fats that we receive from our diet can be grouped into three main categories: unsaturated fats, saturated fats, and trans fats. On the keto diet, you can use unsaturated and saturated fats in the meals that you eat and cook, but you should avoid using any trans fats.

When you include too many trans fats in your diet, such as baked goods, fried foods, hydrogenated vegetable oils, margarine, and ready-made meals, you increase your "bad" low-density lipoprotein (LDL) and decrease your "good" high-density lipoprotein (HDL).

When you consume trans fats, your body is unable to fully absorb these fats, and they accumulate in your blood and arteries. When this happens, your LDL cholesterol becomes elevated. LDL cholesterol can increase your blood pressure because your body has to work harder to pump blood through your body, and both of these factors can contribute to developing heart disease.

To decrease your LDL cholesterol levels, you should cut out trans fats from your diet and switch to healthy fats and oils that can increase your HDL cholesterol levels. HDL helps your body to decrease and protect against LDL cholesterol.

Although you can use saturated fats such as butter, cheese, and heavy cream in your diet, it is suggested that you try to limit them, as they can also elevate your cholesterol levels. Whenever possible, try to replace saturated and trans fats with healthy unsaturated fats, which include avocado, avocado oil, chia seeds, fatty fish, flax seeds, most nuts, olive oil, and olives.

Added Sugars

When you include too much sugar in your diet, triglyceride, which is the type of fat that is found in your bloodstream and tissues, is increased in your body. Your body then uses these triglycerides to provide you with energy when you are not receiving carbohydrates from foods —for example, between meals.

36

If your body is unable to burn this energy, your triglyceride levels will be elevated, which can cause your blood pressure and blood sugar levels to increase. When you continue to expose your body to high levels of triglycerides, you increase your risk of developing type 2 diabetes and heart disease.

When you choose to eat food that contains lots of sugar, your daily calorie intake will be high. If you do not burn off the extra calories in your diet from sugar and you are not active, you can gain weight. Excess weight can also be a contributing factor towards an increased risk in type 2 diabetes and heart disease.

To avoid picking up any additional weight as you turn 50 and older, you should limit the added sugars that you include in your diet and other food items that have a high sugar content. This includes chips, chocolate, desserts, pastries, soda, sweets, and food items that have sugar and sweeteners added to them, such as sweetened dairy products.

Sodium

Sodium is an important nutrient to include in your diet. The average adult aged 50 and older should receive 1,200 to 1,300 mg of sodium in their diet each day at minimum, but not more than 2,300 mg at most. The average American diet often sees people consuming as much as 3,400 mg of sodium each day, and this can be bad for your health.

Many people experience low blood pressure, and they need to include more sodium in their diet, while others experience high blood pressure and are advised to decrease their sodium intake. It is important that you find a balance between the minimum and maximum amounts that works for you and your diet to keep your sodium levels and blood pressure balanced throughout the day.

If you are including too much sodium in your diet, you should check the nutritional information of the foods you are eating and how much sodium they contain. Ready-made meals and processed foods contain high levels of sodium. We also tend to add extra salt and spices to our meals when we do not need to. To decrease your sodium intake, you should choose food options that contain less sodium in them and look at cutting down on how much salt and extra spices you add to your dishes.

Is Keto Right for Me?

A low-carb, high-fat keto diet with a moderate amount of protein is a great option for women who are 50 and older. The keto diet provides a plethora of health benefits and helps to improve current health conditions, such as type 2 diabetes and heart disease.

You might have worries that by consuming so much fat in your diet that it could be unhealthy or that you will gain weight. However, because you are reducing your sugar and carbohydrate intake, your body will need to find a new energy source to provide your body with the energy it needs throughout the day.

Once your body has no more sugar and carbohydrate stores to use as fuel, it will start to burn the fat that you are eating in your diet, and once it has used these fats, it will turn to burning through your body fat to provide your body with energy.

There is also a difference between healthy unsaturated fats and unhealthy saturated and trans fats. With the keto diet, you will be mostly eating healthy unsaturated fats and some saturated fats like cheese and butter, which are significantly healthier than including trans fats in your diet. By reducing your intake of saturated fats and avoiding trans fats, you will actually improve your health, reduce your cholesterol, and be in the best shape of your life.

If you are a vegetarian or a vegan, it is possible for you to follow the keto diet. By eating plant-based foods that are high in fat, such as avocados, coconut oil, nuts, and seeds, you will be able to put your body into ketosis.

You will be able to follow the same food guidelines as one would on the standard low-carb, high-fat keto diet and remove animal products, like dairy, eggs, fish, meat and poultry, seafood, and other animal-based foods like egg white protein, honey, and whey protein. You will only use keto-friendly plant-based ingredients and vegan fortified foods that are keto-friendly.

On a vegetarian or vegan keto diet, you will experience many of the same health benefits as you would if you followed the standard keto diet with animal products included, such as weight loss and reducing your risk of developing type 2 diabetes type 2 and heart disease. You will adopt health benefits gained from following a vegetarian or vegan diet, as well.

If you have an eating disorder, thyroid disease, type 1 diabetes, multiple sclerosis (MS), or have had your gallbladder removed, you should first get the advice of your general practitioner or nutritionist before starting with the keto diet. They will be able to guide you and inform you if there are specific foods or a food group that you need to continue eating that is beneficial to your specific health condition.

Chapter 2: Keto Health Benefits

When you turn 50 and older, you become more concerned with your health and the foods that you are putting into your body. As you age, your metabolism slows down significantly, and you start to lose muscle mass, which causes you to gain weight. With the keto diet, you can improve your health and reduce your risk of developing heart disease, type 2 diabetes, and cancer.

Health Benefits

There are many other health benefits that you can receive from following a keto diet, including:

Reduce Your Appetite and Lose Weight

You can reduce your appetite and lose weight by eating a low-carb keto diet. In fact, in a recent meta-analysis published by the NIH (Mansoor et al., 2016), it was shown that you can lose up to 2 pounds more in a year by following the keto diet when compared to other diets. When you cut out carbohydrates and sugar from your diet and eat more fat and protein, you will find that you do not need to consume as many calories as you would on a nonketo diet and that you feel satiated for longer.

Carbohydrates tend to make you feel bloated and heavy, and they only give your body energy for a short period of time, leaving you exhausted soon after eating them. Low-calorie foods are not only good for you to eat in your 50s to lose excess weight and reduce muscle loss, but they also help your body feel more energized and can reduce water retention and bloating.

Reduce Risk of Heart Disease

Over 647,000 people die from heart disease in America each year. There are various factors that can cause heart disease, such as inflammation in the arteries of the heart, diabetes, cholesterol, high blood pressure, heart defects, smoking, stress, obesity, and not following a well-structured diet.

By eating healthy fats and oils from the keto diet, such as olive oil, you can increase your high-density lipoprotein (HDL) cholesterol and lower your low-density lipoprotein (LDL). HDL is a type of cholesterol that is good for your body and helps to protect against LDL, the unhealthy type of cholesterol. When you eat fats and oils that are bad for you, LDL increases in your bloodstream and can build up in the walls of your arteries. When this happens, you can be at risk of heart disease. Healthy fats and oils help to reduce the LDL and improve your heart health, lowering your risk of developing heart disease.

High blood pressure, otherwise known as hypertension, is one of the main causes of heart disease. When you have high blood pressure, your heart needs to work harder to pump the blood around your body, which can put a strain on your heart. Because of this, your heart can become damaged, and it can progress into heart disease. A low-carb diet can help you to normalize your blood pressure and lower your risk of heart damage and heart disease.

A low-carb, high-fat diet like keto can help you to lose excess weight, feel good about yourself, have lots of energy, and be able to make healthier decisions about your body and nutrition. Weight loss, an exercise routine, and a structured eating plan that caters to your needs as your body ages will help you to reduce your risk of heart disease and help to improve your symptoms if you have developed heart disease.

Improve Type 2 Diabetes

Diabetes is a growing concern worldwide, with over 34 million people in the United States being diabetic. While a low-carb, high-fat diet like keto is not recommended for type 1 diabetics, it can be beneficial for those suffering from type 2 and helps to lower their blood glucose levels. The keto diet can be the healthiest lifestyle change that you can make to reduce your risk of developing type 2 diabetes and manage it effectively if you already suffer from it.

By reducing the number of calories that you consume each day in your diet, losing excess weight, and eating better food choices, you will be able to increase your body's sensitivity to insulin and reduce your blood sugar levels.

Many of the foods in the keto diet have a low glycemic load. This means that your blood sugar will not suddenly spike by eating these foods, compared to if you ate foods that contain a high glycemic load. By eating foods with a low glycemic load, you can stabilize your blood sugar and reduce your body's need for insulin.

When you reduce your carbohydrates and increase your intake of fat, your body creates ketones to process these fats into a source of energy that your body can use throughout the day. The process that your body goes through to create these ketones helps to improve your response and resistance to insulin.

Reduce Risk of Cancer

The keto diet can help reduce your risk of developing cancer and is often used hand-in-hand with cancer treatment to help improve your symptoms if you are already suffering from cancer.

It has been found that some tumors grow larger and can spread in the presence of glucose sugar. By restricting carbohydrates and sugar in your diet, you can reduce the growth of these cancerous growths and stop them from spreading further.

If you are suffering from cancer, you should talk to your general practitioner or nutritionist before starting the keto diet so that you can get their advice and they can potentially monitor your cancerous cell growth while you are on the keto diet.

Improve Brain Disorders

The keto diet first came about as a diet to help treat children who were suffering from epilepsy and other brain disorders. Over the years, people have found that the keto diet can not only just work for children but also for people of all ages, including those in their 50s or older.

When carbohydrates and sugars are removed from a person's diet and their fat intake increases, their body is unable to use either as an energy source, and their body and brain uses ketones to burn the fat that they consume from their diet to give them energy throughout the day. When this happens, the person's brain receives energy from the ketones that are produced in their body and as a result they experience fewer seizures.

The keto diet can also be beneficial to people who are suffering from Alzheimer's and Parkinson's disease. It has been shown that by eating a keto diet, you can decrease the symptoms associated with Alzheimer's disease and stop it from getting worse. Symptoms of Parkinson's disease can also be improved with the keto diet.

Improve Symptoms of PCOS

Polycystic ovary syndrome (PCOS) is a health condition whereby a woman's body produces more male hormones than it normally should. When this happens, you might experience irregular or skipped periods, and you will have problems with getting pregnant. If you have PCOS, you have a higher risk of heart disease and developing type 2 diabetes.

When you eat foods that contain carbohydrates and sugar, your insulin levels increase. When your insulin levels are high and you suffer from PCOS, your ovaries produce male hormones like testosterone, which in turn can cause your periods to become more irregular and cause you to grow more body hair.

By following a low-carb, high-fat keto diet, your insulin levels will remain steady and, as a result, your ovaries will not produce more male hormones in your body than it needs. This allows your period to become more regular and helps to improve other symptoms related to PCOS that you might be experiencing.

Improve Symptoms of Metabolic Syndrome

When you are at risk of developing type 2 diabetes and heart disease, you will experience symptoms, called metabolic syndrome, which include gaining weight around your stomach area, your levels of "good" HDL cholesterol have decreased and your "bad" LDL cholesterol has increased, high blood pressure, high blood sugar levels, and an increased amount of triglycerides in your blood.

By following a low-carb, high fat keto diet, you will be able to treat and even reverse these symptoms and improve your quality of life by decreasing your risk of developing type 2 diabetes and heart disease. The keto diet can help you to lose stomach weight, improve your levels of "good" HDL cholesterol, stabilize your blood pressure and blood sugar levels, and decrease the triglycerides in your blood.

Menopause

The keto diet can be beneficial to women at the age of 50 and older who are going through menopause. There are three phases of menopause that all women go through, which are perimenopause, menopause, and postmenopause. You are considered postmenopausal when you have not had a period in over 12 months.

Most women go through menopause in their late 40s to early 50s, but not all women experience it at the same age as other women, and you might find that you have gone through menopause early or that you are yet to go through menopause.

When you start menopause will depend on various factors, such as when other women in your family like your mother, sister, or grandmother experienced menopause, whether you use oral contraceptives or not, your weight, how many pregnancies you have had, whether you smoke or drink alcohol, and whether you are physically active or not.

Perimenopause is the phase you go through before you become menopausal and usually begins when you are in your mid to late 40s. When you go through perimenopause, your body will go through new changes, and you will start to experience various symptoms such as hot flashes, being unable to sleep at night or being restless during the night, feeling lethargic, vaginal dryness, breaking into hot sweats in the night, not being able to remember things or struggling to focus, and having mood swings.

These symptoms are usually the worst in the perimenopause phase and continue on into the menopause and postmenopause stage. However, many women who do not experience these symptoms severely in the perimenopausal stage might find that these symptoms worsen in the later menopausal and postmenopausal phases.

When a woman becomes perimenopausal, her estrogen and progesterone levels in her body decrease. Estrogen and progesterone are hormones that are used in a woman's body to help support the functioning of the reproductive system and to keep a woman's menstrual cycle regular. When these hormones decrease, your reproductive system will release fewer eggs, and your menstrual cycle will no longer be regular.

When you were younger, the estrogen hormone would work to distribute your stored fat into your hips and thighs. However, as you become older and your estrogen decreases, this fat is redirected to your stomach area. When fat stores in your stomach area, you become more at risk of developing heart disease, insulin resistance, and type 2 diabetes.

With this decrease in estrogen levels, along with an increase in the ghrelin hormone, which is responsible for your feeling of hunger, you will find that your appetite and cravings will be increased, causing you to eat more food and gain weight at a faster rate than before you started menopause.

Other hormones that change during menopause and muscle loss that occurs as you turn 50 and older can also act against you during this time and make it easy to gain weight. A low-carb keto diet can help you manage your weight more effectively, decrease the amount of weight that you gain, and help you to get rid of food cravings.

With the reduction of estrogen in the body and removing energy sources like sugar and carbohydrates from your diet, your body and brain will create ketones that will use the fat that you consume from the keto diet as an alternative source of energy. Your hot flashes stem from receiving glucose in your brain, and when your brain no longer receives glucose from your diet, the severity and frequency of hot flashes that you experience is reduced. The keto diet has also been found to improve your mood and protect your memory against remembering things and improve your concentration.

It is suggested that when you follow the keto diet and you are going through menopause that you should further restrict your carbohydrate intake from the allowed 50 grams per day to between 20 to 30 grams per day so that your body goes into ketosis and can successfully help to relieve these symptoms.

Chapter 3: Starting the Keto Diet

So, you have taken into consideration how your body is changing and the nutrients that you will need as you turn 50 and older. You have also gone through the health benefits, and you feel that the keto diet is the perfect fit for you. That is wonderful! Now it is time for you to take the first steps towards starting the keto diet and identifying which foods you will be eating and which you should be avoiding.

Food Guidelines

The keto diet can appear to be quite complicated and possibly daunting at first glance when you see all the foods you can eat and which you should not. As a general rule of thumb, you should focus on increasing your consumption of healthy fatty foods, with a moderate amount of protein, while cutting out sugars and carbs.

I have provided a comprehensive list below of all the foods that you are allowed to eat and the ones that should be restricted and avoided. When you first start cooking with keto-friendly ingredients, I suggest that you keep a list of them somewhere you can see them so that you can easily refer back to it if there is something you are unsure of.

Once you start cooking keto, you will begin to see how easy it is, and you will quickly grasp an understanding of which foods are keto and which are not without having to refer back to your list as frequently.

Here is a list of all of the foods that you can include in the keto diet, with some extra foods that have very low amounts of carbs in them that you can include now and again with your meals. However, you should always moderate how much of these you eat and try to aim to include foods that contain less than 5% carbs.

- **Berries.** When you choose berries, you should look for ones that do not contain much sugar, such as blackberries, blueberries, and raspberries. They make great snacks, but you should limit yourself to small amounts at a time because they contain sugar and carbs.
- **Beverages.** There are a few different beverages that you can include on the keto diet, including bone broth, unsweetened coffee and tea, and water. If you feel like switching things up with water, you can try

a water infusion. For this, you should get a fusion bottle, and then cut up some lemon, lime, or cucumber and add it into the middle section. You can add these fruits to your water to give them different flavors that get stronger throughout the day.

- **Dairy.** You can use high-fat dairy products to create creamy and delicious foods. Dairy products that you can add to your diet include butter, cream cheese, cottage cheese, heavy cream, plain Greek yogurt, sour cream, and unprocessed hard and soft cheeses. Milk often contains sugars in it, so it is recommended that you switch your milk out for cream.

- **Fats and oils.** With the keto diet, healthy fats and oils will become an essential source of energy for your body to go into ketosis and lose weight. Seventy to eighty percent of your diet should contain healthy fats and oils, and the best way to incorporate them into your meals is to cook with them. Fats and oils that you can use include avocado oil, butter, cocoa butter, coconut butter, coconut oil, eggs, ghee, lard, olive oil, macadamia oil, mayonnaise, MCT oil, and tallow.

- **Fish and seafood.** Fish, shellfish, and other seafood are high in healthy fats and oils. You can include all types of fish, shellfish, and seafood into your diet, such as catfish, clams, cod, crab, halibut, lobster, mussels, oysters, salmon, scallops, snapper, trout, and tuna.

- **Meat.** It is suggested that when you buy meat that you should choose ones that are unprocessed, such as bacon, chicken, ground beef, ham, lamb, pork, steak, and turkey. You should try to avoid processed meat, such as cold meats, meatballs, and sausages, as much as possible because they tend to contain hidden carbs that are added in the meat production process. If you want to eat processed meat, you should limit yourself and make sure that it contains less than 5% carbs.

- **Nuts and seeds.** Another great source of healthy fats and oils comes from unsalted nuts and seeds. They work well for snacks and as toppings on your meals. However, you should try to moderate how many nuts you have, as they can contain carbs. You can include most nuts and seeds into your keto diet, such as almonds, Brazil nuts, chia seeds, flax seed, macadamia nuts, pecan nuts, pumpkin seeds, sesame seeds, and walnuts.

- **Herbs and spices.** Some keto-friendly herbs and spices that do not contain a lot of carbs in them include basil, cayenne pepper, chili powder, cilantro, cinnamon, cumin, garlic powder, oregano, parsley, rosemary, and thyme.
- **Sweeteners.** You can include sweeteners like stevia and sucralose into your tea and coffee now and again if you do not really drink much of these beverages. However, they can be unhealthy for you, and you should try limiting this as much as possible.
- **Vegetables.** When choosing vegetables to add to your dishes, you should choose ones that grow above the ground and those which are nonstarchy. These include asparagus, cauliflower, cucumber, eggplants, garlic, green beans, mushrooms, olives, onions, peppers, tomatoes, and zucchini, as well as leafy greens

like broccoli, brussels sprouts, cabbage, kale, lettuce, and spinach.

Here is a list of the foods that you should restrict or try to avoid in your diet. When you remove these foods from your diet, your body will be able to cycle into ketosis, and you will be able to meet your weight loss goals.

If you are struggling to lose weight following the keto diet, then you may need to refer back to this list to see if any foods you are eating are included or if you are eating too many food sources that contain sugar and carbs.

- **Alcohol.** All types of alcohol should be avoided because they contain sugar and carbohydrates. This includes beer, cider, wine, and other alcoholic drinks that have been sweetened like cocktails.
- **Condiments.** Store-bought condiments contain sugar and

should be avoided. If you would like to use condiments, I suggest that you make them yourself using keto recipes. This way, you know exactly what you are putting into them, and there are no added sugars like you would find in bottled condiments.

- **Fruits.** Fruits contain high amounts of sugar in them, so they should be avoided. Most fruits should be avoided, unless they contain low amounts of sugar in them. This includes apples, bananas, cherries, dried fruits, fruit juices, grapefruit, grapes, mangos, melon, nectarines, oranges, peaches, pears, pineapple, plums, smoothies made from fruit, tangerines, and watermelon.
- **Grains.** You will find that most of the carbohydrates you eat come from grains. All grains, including whole grains, should be

avoided when following the keto diet. These grains include amaranth, barley, buckwheat, bulgur, flour and corn tortillas, millet, oatmeal, oats, pumpernickel, quinoa, rice, rye, sandwich wraps, sorghum, sourdough, sprouted grains, and wheat.

- **Legumes.** Another food group that you should avoid that is high in carbohydrates is legumes. This includes black beans, cannellini, chickpeas, kidney beans, lentils, navy beans, pinto beans, and soybeans.
- **Low-fat dairy.** Any low-fat dairy products should be avoided, and you should swap any of these out for alternatives with higher fat content. This includes fat-free yogurt, low-fat cheese, skim milk, and skim mozzarella.
- **Starchy vegetables.** Most vegetables are fine to eat, but

others contain high amounts of carbohydrates. Like with grains and legumes, you should try to avoid eating starchy vegetables in your diet. Starchy vegetables include artichokes, butternut squash, corn, parsnips, peas, potatoes, sweet potatoes, and yams.

- **Sugar.** All forms of sugars and sweeteners that are not stevia and sucralose should be avoided. This includes agave nectar, aspartame, cane sugar, corn syrup, honey, maple syrup, saccharin, and Splenda.
- **Sweet treats.** Because sweet treats and baked goods often contain high levels of sugar, you should avoid buying these from the store. If you are craving something sweet, you can look at a few keto dessert recipes and make yourself a few snacks and

treats according to the list of allowed keto-friendly foods.

- **Trans fats and oils.** Any fats and oils that contain trans fats are bad for your health and should be avoided. You can swap these trans fats and oils out for the healthy fats and oils on the list of allowed foods. Fats and oils that contain trans fats include canola oil, grapeseed oil, margarine, peanut oil, sesame oil, soybean oil, and sunflower oil.

You should remember that you are not completely cutting out foods that contain carbohydrates with the keto diet. When you first start with the keto diet, you should begin with eating 20 grams of carbohydrates each day so that you can put your body into ketosis. You should continue with this amount to lose weight and meet your health goals before you start introducing more carbs into your diet.

When you are choosing foods that contain carbohydrates, you should ensure that their net carbs are less than 5 grams. How this works is that if you have a food item with total carbs equaling 5 grams, you then check how much fiber it contains. If, for example, the food item contains 2 grams of fiber, then you will subtract that from the total carbs. In this example, your net carbs will be equal to 3 grams.

You will use the net carb amount to keep track of how many carbs you are including in your diet. You should do this for each food item that you will be eating that contains some carbohydrates in it until you reach your maximum daily allowance of 20 grams.

Once you are ready to bring your body out of ketosis, then you can increase your carbohydrate intake to between 20 to 50 grams per day.

How to Start the Keto Diet

To start a keto diet, you first need to become accustomed to the foods you will be eating and the ones you will be restricting and avoiding. You could make photocopies of the food guidelines I provided earlier and put them up onto your fridge, or you could take pictures on your phone to refer back to, whichever suits you best.

Decide on a Start Date

When you have decided that you want to follow the keto diet, you should decide on a date that you want to start and commit to it. By deciding on a start date, you can give yourself time to prepare mentally, sit down with your family to discuss whether you will be doing the keto diet alone or if someone wants to do it with you, and get all the foods and ingredients that you will need for the diet.

I suggest that you start the diet during a time when you do not have any commitments or events coming up, like a birthday party or a wedding, where you will feel obligated to eat foods that are not within the keto diet's guidelines. If you are unable to avoid this type of thing, then you should either readjust your start date to another date or try your best to stick to the keto diet with the foods that they serve you.

However, if you choose the second option, there is a possibility that you may not have lost as much weight as you were expecting to when you weigh yourself again, but you should try not to be discouraged and pick up where you left off after the event. If you ate too many carbohydrates on the day of the event, you should try and consume very little to no carbohydrates the next day so that you can kickstart your body back into ketosis.

Ideally, you should pick a start date where you can dedicate your time to learning about keto-friendly foods and how to cook and experiment with them, and also one when you know you are not going to be doing strenuous activities so that when you get the keto flu, you can take it easy and work through it until it passes.

Organize Your Food Cupboards

Before you start with the keto diet, I suggest that you have a look at what foods are in your cupboards and see what you can still use and what you cannot. I suggest that you rid your cupboards of items that have a high content of sugar, and grains, and starchy vegetables to begin with. Make sure that you go according to the food guidelines at the beginning of this chapter when deciding what can stay and what should go. By doing this, you can remove any temptation and start the keto diet with a clean slate.

However, this is not always an option if you live with other people who are not going to be following the same diet as you. In this case, I suggest that you either try and separate the foods in the cupboard from the foods that you will be using for the keto diet so that you do not use something that you should avoid by mistake, or you can try and go through everything and take note of which foods have high sugar or carbohydrate contents so that you know which foods to avoid when you are cooking.

Transitioning to Keto

There is no one way that you should use to transition to the keto diet. We all adapt to a new lifestyle change in different ways, and what works for you might not work for someone else. It is important that you find a method that suits you and your current lifestyle and that you start working toward your goals.

Here are a few of the most common ways that you can transition to the keto diet:

- **Going cold turkey.** Sometimes cutting out all of the foods that you should be avoiding is the best method to get started with the keto diet. Like ripping off a Band-Aid, the worst part about any diet is the first few days after you have started. If you approach the keto diet in a cold turkey method, you will be able to get over the worst of the cravings and keto flu (which we will discuss in detail later in this chapter) quickly and be able to enjoy everything that the keto diet has to offer sooner.

- **One food group at a time.** Another approach you can use is by starting to cut out one food group at a time over the course of a few days or a few weeks. The first day you can remove sugar from your diet, and the next carbs, and so on, until you have removed all food groups or specific foods that you should avoid on the keto diet. This method can help you ease into the diet and find alternatives for the foods you love as you cut them out one-by-one.

- **One meal at a time.** If cutting out food groups one at a time is not right for you, but neither is going cold turkey, you can try to make one meal a day that is keto for a few days or weeks instead, and then add in a second meal when you are ready, and so on, until you are only eating keto foods for all of your meals. With this method, you can take your time learning specific recipes for each meal of the day and get used to cooking them as you ease yourself into the keto diet.

- **Carb reduction.** If the above transition methods are not working for you, you can try the carb reduction method. How this works is you will start out with eating carbs like you would with a standard nonketo diet, and then you will reduce the carbs from your meals slowly until you are eating the recommended keto amount to put your body into ketosis. For example, you will start out with 250 grams of carbohydrates per day, and the next day 200 grams of carbohydrates, and so on, until you are only including 20 grams of carbohydrates in your diet each day. With this method, you can go as slowly or as quickly as you want, whichever makes you most comfortable.

Use a Tracking App for the Foods You Eat

When you start with the keto diet, you should download a tracking app to keep track of the foods that you are eating and the specific nutrients that you are receiving from those foods. You will need to ensure that you choose a tracking app that tracks your protein, fat, and carbohydrate intake from the foods you eat.

An application that I like to use is the MyFitnessPal application. In the app, you can select the food item that you are eating or the ingredients you have included in a meal. It also lets you choose the size and quantity of the food item used, for example, one cup of diced onions. There is also an option you can use to scan the barcode of specific food items that you can quickly add to your food list. MyFitnessPal gives you all the nutritional information that you need to know, such as how much sugar or sodium is in a food item.

There are also many other applications that you can use to track this type of information. You should have a look and explore which applications work for you. These applications give you a good indication of whether you are eating the right amounts of proteins, fats, and carbohydrates, and you can also check the nutritional information of food that you want to make to ensure it falls within your daily allowance.

Prepare for the Keto Flu

When you start the keto diet for the first time, you will experience "keto flu" symptoms, such as feeling nauseated, having severe cravings for sugary foods, experiencing muscle pains and cramps, headaches, feeling dizzy, struggling to concentrate, and feeling moody and irritable. Everyone will experience some measure of keto flu symptoms when they first start keto, whether you have done the keto diet before or not.

However, if you are experiencing severe keto flu symptoms, you should first look at trying a different keto diet transition method. For example, if you are going cold turkey, then it might not be the right approach for you, and you should choose a way to transition that will ease you into it a bit more slowly.

You might also be transitioning into the keto diet too fast. In this case, you

82

should slow down and take a step back. For example, if you are cutting out one food group a day, you should space it out a bit more instead and look at cutting out a food group every second day, or even once a week. It does not matter how quickly you are transitioning into the diet. What matters more is that you are following the keto diet the correct way and eating the right foods, not to mention that you are enjoying the journey along the way.

Another reason why you might be experiencing keto flu is because you might not be consuming enough fat in your diet. When you are following a low-carb, high-fat diet, you need to replace your carbohydrate energy source with fat. If you are not receiving enough needed fat in your diet throughout the day, then your body is unable to provide you with enough of an energy source and will need to work harder to burn your fat storage instead. You should ensure that you have enough fat in your diet throughout the day to help alleviate keto flu symptoms.

When you are experiencing keto flu symptoms, your body and muscles will feel weaker, and you will have aches and pains. During this time, I suggest that you take it easy and do not perform strenuous activities and intensive workout routines, as this can make your keto flu symptoms feel worse. However, you should continue to keep active with some light exercise, such as walking or yoga, to ensure that you are meeting your maximum weight loss potential while your body is in ketosis.

When you start the keto diet, you will notice that you are losing a lot of weight. But a lot of the weight you lose will be from water retention in your body. This can cause you to become dehydrated, and you might feel dizzy and confused and struggle to concentrate. To combat dehydration, you should ensure that you remain hydrated and take electrolytes if you need to.

Ketosis

When you eat a low-carb, high-fat keto diet, your body will go into a state of ketosis, where it will switch from using carbohydrates and sugar as a source of energy to using ketones which act to burn the fat that you consume from the diet instead. To put your body into ketosis, you should ensure that you are eating fewer than 50 grams of carbohydrates each day.

The process of putting your body into a ketosis state does not happen immediately, and it can take a while before your body adapts to the changes. It can take two to seven days before your body goes into ketosis. The rate at which you go into ketosis depends on various factors, including what your body type is, how many carbs you are eating each day, and how active you are.

You can decrease the time it takes for your body to go into ketosis by decreasing your carbohydrate intake to under 20 grams, by supplementing certain nutrients in your diet, and doing intermittent fasting, where you only eat between certain times in the day.

So, how do I know if I am in ketosis, you ask? You will notice various indicators when your body has gone into ketosis, including weight loss, increased energy, reduced appetite, bad breath, improved focus and concentration, problems with your digestion like constipation and diarrhea, and not being able to sleep.

There are specialized ketone analyzer devices that you can buy that can help you monitor whether you are in ketosis or not. This is a great tool that you can use to give you accurate readings, although it can be quite pricey. You can use a blood ketone meter to measure the ketone levels in your blood, and it is the most accurate form of testing you can perform. You can also use a ketone breath analyzer to measure the ketone levels in your breath. This method is not as accurate as testing your blood, but it is also still quite accurate.

Going into ketosis can have some adverse side effects, such as feeling tired, constipation, headache, bad breath, and increased levels of cholesterol, but these symptoms do not last throughout the entirety of the period that you are in ketosis, and these symptoms should go away after a while. After these initial symptoms, you will find that ketosis is relatively safe for your health and does not impact it negatively.

While staying in ketosis does not pose a problem to your health, you should come out of ketosis once you have reached your health and weight loss goals. It is recommended that you come out of ketosis every three months, if you have not already come out of it sooner.

If your body goes out of ketosis before you have reached your health and weight loss goals, then you might not be following the keto diet in the right way, or you are including too many carbohydrates in your diet. When this happens, you can put your body back into ketosis by doing the same things you did the first time.

Shopping List

Going to the shops and buying groceries and produce for a new diet can be tricky when you are not sure what you should be buying and how much of each you should get. With a weekly shopping list,

you do not need to worr
are going to start your di
are going to do, and in
focus on what really ma
getting the food you need
and cooking delicious keto

As you continue on your keto journey, you will develop your own preferences, and you might chop and change things from this original shopping list, which is great. Everyone has different tastes. You might find that you do not like something and prefer not to buy it, or you might find a food you enjoy incorporating into many of your dishes.

I encourage you to use this shopping list as a starting point and turn it into a shopping list that works for you to make the most of your keto diet.

Dairy:

- cottage cheese
- cream cheese
- hard cheeses

- heavy cream
- plain Greek yogurt
- soft cheeses

Nuts:

- almonds
- brazil nuts
- hazelnuts
- macadamia nuts
- pecan nuts
- walnuts

Fats and Oils:

- almond butter
- avocado oil
- butter
- coconut butter
- coconut oil
- duck
- ghee
- hazelnut oil
- mayonnaise
- lard
- MCT oil
- olive oil

- olives
- sesame oil
- tallow

Fruits:

- blackberries
- blueberries
- coconut
- lemon
- lime
- raspberries
- strawberries
- tomato
- watermelon

Pantry Items:

- almond flour
- beef broth
- bone broth
- chicken broth
- coconut flour
- coffee
- herbal tea
- stevia

Protein:

- bacon
- beef
- chicken
- eggs
- fish
- ham
- organ meats
- pork
- salmon
- sardines
- steak
- tuna
- turkey

Seeds:

- chia seeds
- flax seeds
- pumpkin seeds

Vegetables:

- asparagus
- avocado
- bell pepper

- broccoli
- brussels sprouts
- cabbage
- cauliflower
- celery
- cucumber
- eggplant
- garlic
- green beans
- jalapeño peppers
- lettuce
- kale
- mushrooms
- spinach
- tomatoes
- zucchini

Chapter 4: Easy Keto Substitutes

What makes a diet difficult is knowing that you cannot eat the foods that you used to be able to eat or cook with your favorite ingredients. But that does not have to be the case when you follow the keto diet. Along with all the foods that you can eat on the keto diet, like protein and fats, there are also some simple substitutes that you can include in your diet.

Food Swaps

Below I have listed all of the food swaps that you can make on the keto diet and what goes well in place of foods that you have removed from your diet:

Bread and Wraps

While high-carb bread and wraps are off the menu with the keto diet, it does not mean that you cannot make your own low-carb substitutes that are keto friendly. You can use various keto-friendly flours in your cooking to make bread, taco shells, tortilla chips, and tortillas. Flours that are low-carb and keto friendly include almond flour, coconut flour, ground flax, low-carb almond meal or ground almonds, and psyllium husk. You should ensure that you have these flours in your food cupboard so that you can make breads and wraps whenever you need them.

However, if you are trying to avoid eating carbohydrates completely in your diet, you could use chard, collard, or lettuce instead. Iceberg or romaine lettuce works well to wrap around burger patties to keep them together and can also be used as a substitute for wraps and taco shells. You can also chard and collard as a substitute for hand rolls, unwiches, and wraps.

Similar to chard, but which is much thinner, nori sheets can be used as a substitute for wraps and hand rolls to hold the contents together. You can also use nori sheets when making your own keto-friendly sushi to hold cauliflower rice or Shirataki rice mixed with cream cheese or keto-friendly mayonnaise. Yum!

Breading

Breadcrumbs can help to bring out the flavor in your food and can add a new texture to it. Breading also works well to coat meat when you bake or barbecue it, as a coating for chicken nuggets and strips, or even for use as the outer coating of filled cheese balls. However, breadcrumbs can be high in carbs, and you therefore cannot include them in your diet. Other alternative low-carb options that you can use instead of breadcrumbs are almond flour, crushed chicken crackling, crushed pork rinds, flaxseeds, and shredded parmesan cheese. You should make your own chicken crackling and pork rinds, if possible, so that you can ensure that there is no added sugar or carbohydrates that go into the process.

Cereals

If you want to add more variety to your breakfast meals, you can make your own low-carb granola cereal. By adding a granola mix to your food cupboard, you can have more of a breakfast selection for when you are on-the-go and do not have time to make yourself something in the morning.

To make your granola mix, you can use a mix of chia seeds, coconut chips, flaked almonds, and hemp seeds. You can also use other low-carb keto-friendly seeds and nuts to your liking. You can store your granola mix in an airtight container in your food cupboard and serve on top of full-fat plain Greek yogurt or a milk substitute, such as almond milk, that does not contain any added sugars and that has not been sweetened. You can top with a few low-carb berries, like blackberries, blueberries, and raspberries.

High-Carb Fruits

When you are following the keto diet, you should avoid all fruits that are high in sugar and carbohydrates. However, there are a few options such as avocado, berries, coconut, rhubarb, and watermelon that you can still include in your diet that are low-carb options. Berries that you can use include blackberries, blueberries, raspberries, and strawberries.

You should try to limit your intake of these fruits, but they can be added to your cooking and baking to give it a burst of flavor and sweetness. Some fruits can increase your blood sugar levels, so you should keep an eye on this when you include these fruits in your diet, and if something spikes your blood sugar levels, then you might need to avoid it.

Legumes

Some low-carb nuts like peanuts and macadamia nuts can be used in your meals to add flavor in place of legumes like beans, lentils, and chickpeas, which are high in carbs. If you usually add chickpeas or beans to your salads, you can swap these out for peanuts and macadamia nuts, or cashews if you do not mind a higher carb count. These nuts can also work well to add as toppings to your foods.

If you like to use hummus as a dip with snacks or if you are having a Mediterranean night, you can use macadamia nuts as a substitute to using chickpeas and crush them to create a keto-friendly hummus paste.

While you can use nuts as toppings on your meals, it does not work that well when adding them to some meals like soups and stews. In this case, you can replace the beans and lentils that you would add to your meals with vegetables that are low in carbohydrates, like eggplant and green beans.

Milk

Asking whether you can include milk in your baking, cooking, or beverages is not a question that can easily be answered. Most milk that is sold at the grocery stores is packed full of added sugars and carbohydrates. Wherever possible, you should choose unsweetened milk options, such as almond milk, cashew milk, coconut milk, and flax milk.

When you buy milk, you should check the sugar and carbohydrate nutritional information on the label. You should make sure that any milk that you buy is full fat. However, it is suggested that you switch out all your milk in your food and beverages to a heavy cream option because it contains no added sugars or carbohydrates in it.

When you buy yogurt, you should switch out the one you usually buy with unsweetened plain yogurt or plain Greek yogurt that does not have added sugars or carbohydrates. Not everyone likes plain yogurt, but you can add toppings like chia seeds, coconut butter, nuts, and spices to give it more flavor.

Pasta

A great food swap for pasta and spaghetti is to use low-carb vegetable noodles. You can use any nonstarchy vegetables, such as celery, cucumber, rutabaga, turnips, and zucchini, and cut them lengthwise into thin strips with a sharp knife, or you can use a spiralizer tool to help you achieve this. You should also be able to find precut vegetable noodles from the grocery store.

Once you have sliced the noodles, you can add them into a greased pan and cook them for one to three minutes. They cook faster than carbohydrate-loaded noodles, and you can add protein and toppings the way you normally would.

If you have tried vegetable noodles, and they do not appeal to you, then you can try Shirataki noodles, which are created by crushing the Japanese konjac plant and forming it into different pasta variations, such as fettuccine, noodles, rice, and spaghetti. Shirataki noodles have no carbohydrates and are extremely low in calories. Various Shirataki noodle brands are sold on Amazon.

Kelp noodles are a similar option to Shirataki noodles that you can try. You can eat these noodles raw, or you can make them soft in boiling water or by adding them to soup to serve with one of your meals, such as a spaghetti bolognaise. You can also buy these noodles on Amazon.

Potatoes

Potatoes are versatile and can be incorporated into every meal by boiling, frying, mashing, or roasting them, but they contain high amounts of carbohydrates and are not keto friendly. Potato substitutes that you can use on the keto diet include cauliflower, celery, kohlrabi, radishes, rutabaga, and turnips.

Cauliflower can be used to make a mash that you can use as a side to your keto meals. To make cauliflower mash, you will need to take a head of cauliflower and cut out the stem and remove the leaves. Next, you will cut the cauliflower into florets and put them into a food processor. You should process a few florets at a time, and then add some water or heavy cream and butter to the processed florets. Then, you should continue to process the mixture until it forms a smooth puree. Scoop out the puree and set aside in a separate dish, and continue to do this until all the florets have been processed.

To make fries and snacks, you should try a variety of different ingredients and see which work the best with what you are trying to make. If you want to make substitute potato fries, you can use rutabaga, which gives the fries a similar taste and texture to potato fries. If you want to make substitute crisps, you can use rutabaga and slice it into thin strips. You can also use low-carb vegetables like eggplant, mushrooms, and zucchini.

Rice

Cauliflower is low carb, it has great taste, and can be used to replace high-carb foods like couscous, rice, and risotto. It is a versatile ingredient that mixes together well with many other foods and gives good texture to your meals. You can either buy cauliflower rice premade in the grocery store, or you can make it yourself. You can also use broccoli and celery to make cauliflower rice, instead of cauliflower, if you do not like the taste or you want to try something new.

To make your own cauliflower rice, you will need to take a head of cauliflower and cut out the stem and remove the leaves. Next, you will cut the cauliflower into florets and put the florets into a food processor. Process the florets until the granules are about the size of rice, and do not overprocess it. You can also use the food processor's grating blade to do this, if it has one. Then you can simply add the cauliflower rice to your meal and enjoy.

Another low-carb option that you can use for rice in your meals is Shirataki rice. Like Shirataki noodles, Shirataki rice is also created by crushing the

Japanese konjac plant, but instead of forming noodles from the konjac mixture, they made rice grains instead. Shirataki rice has fewer carbohydrates in it than cauliflower rice and can be used to ensure you are eating as few carbohydrates as possible to keep you in ketosis. Cauliflower rice and Shirataki rice go well together and can be combined if you are looking for a different taste in your rice.

You can use both cauliflower rice and Shirataki rice to make sushi by using cream cheese or some keto-friendly homemade mayonnaise to make the rice sticky.

Sugar and Syrups

While it is not recommended that you include sweeteners often in your cooking, baking, and beverages because it is not good for your health in the long term, you can use them in the keto diet as a substitute for sugar. Sweeteners that are keto friendly are erythritol, monk fruit, stevia, and xylitol. These sweeteners work well with the keto diet because they do not raise your blood pressure and do not contain any calories.

You can use as much sweetener as you need to so that you can make your food and beverages to your tastes, but they can be bitter and taste artificial if you use too much. You should not include sweeteners in your diet that will raise your blood sugar, such as sweeteners with dextrose and maltodextrin in them.

In addition, you can use xylitol syrup and yacon syrup in your cooking, baking, and beverages. Yacon syrup is quite popular because it has a low glycemic load, does not raise your blood pressure, and has many health benefits, such as helping you lose weight by reducing your appetite if taken before a meal, reducing your risk of developing cancer, improving your bone health, improving your immune system to help fight against bacteria and infections, improving your insulin resistance, and improving digestion.

Vegetable Oils

Vegetable fats and oils, such as canola oil, corn oil, grapeseed oil, margarine, peanut oil, rapeseed oil, safflower oil, and soybean oil, are high in unhealthy trans fats that are bad for your health and can increase your "bad" LDL cholesterol levels.

When you are following the keto diet, you should ensure that you are substituting these fats with healthier options, which are saturated and unsaturated fats.

Saturated fats can be heated and are mostly used when you start cooking. Saturated fats that you should include in your cooking instead of using vegetable oils include butter, coconut oil, ghee, lard, MCT oil, and tallow. If possible, you should switch out your cooking oils for MCT oil instead, which aids in digestion and is recommended on the keto diet because it is transferred directly into ketones that your body can use.

Meanwhile, unsaturated fats should be for cold use and are usually added when you are finished cooking. Unsaturated fats that you can add to your cooking as a substitute to vegetable oils include avocado oil, macadamia nut oil, and olive oil.

Wheat Flour

When you remove high-carb flours and wheats from your diet, you might feel that you are limited to what you can cook and bake. However, you will still have low-carb flour substitutes that you can use to make breads, wraps, and baked goods. Flours that are low in carbs and keto-friendly include almond flour, coconut flour, flaxseed powder, and psyllium powder.

These substitutes will still contain carbohydrates but will have significantly less than when eating foods that have nonketo flours in them. Wherever possible, you should try to cut out the bread and flours that you use, even if it is keto-friendly, because a high carb content can take your body out of ketosis, and you will not lose as much weight as you were expecting. You should instead try to replace breads with other keto substitutes such as lettuce to keep a sandwich together so that you can ensure that you lose the weight that you should when your body is in ketosis.

If you are feeling like you are in the mood to make pizza, you can ditch the flour and other wheats and use cauliflower instead to form a pizza dough that you can roll out and add toppings to. Toppings you can include on a pizza that are keto-friendly include nonstarchy vegetables like cucumbers, olives, onions, peppers, and tomatoes, and you can top with various cheeses, such as mozzarella and parmesan cheese. You should experiment with various toppings and see which you like. I always enjoy putting ground beef on mine and topping with mozzarella and parmesan cheese when I make pizza.

However, when baking and making sweet treats, there are not many other options than to include these flours into your baked goods. To increase the amount of fat that you are receiving from your baked goods and to make them more keto friendly, you can substitute avocado into your baking instead of using oil and butter. You might be worried that this will change the flavor of your baking into something more savory, but you will be pleasantly surprised by the richness of your baking when you add it in.

Reading Nutritional Information

You might have been asking yourself how you can tell if a food item is keto friendly or not. You can check this by looking at the nutritional label on the back of the item.

First, you should go through the ingredients listed on the label and see which ones are mentioned first and which are mentioned last. If an ingredient is mentioned first in the list, then there is more of that one ingredient than the others that come after it in the list. If starch or sugar is mentioned in the first five ingredients, then it is most likely not a keto-friendly ingredient, as it will contain high levels of carbohydrates and sugar.

Second, you should calculate the net carbs that are contained in the food item. To do this, you will take the total carbohydrates, for example 4 grams, and subtract the dietary fiber, for example 1 gram, and if there are any sugar alcohols, then you should also subtract those. This will give you the net carbs for a specific food item, which will be 3 grams as per the example used. You should ensure that you keep your net carbs under 5 grams per food item that you eat.

Third, if you are eating food items from a larger pack, you should check what the nutritional information is for a single serving size and how large that serving size is. This will give you the information that you need to make an informed decision about how much you can have while you are following the keto diet. For example, if you have bought a 32 oz packet of almond nuts and a single serving size is indicated to be 1 oz, which is 23 almond nuts, then there are 32 servings in the packet. The net carbohydrate count for 1 oz of almond nuts is 2.6 grams.

Chapter 5: Basic Keto Recipes to Get Started

The hardest part about starting any new diet is learning how to cook with and incorporate ingredients that you do not usually cook with in ways that will make your meals taste delicious.

Many people tend to have difficulties with this part of the diet because they are uncertain about what foods they should be eating and include foods in their meals that they should be avoiding or limiting, and they become frustrated and do not understand why they are not meeting their diet goals. As a result, they give up on the diet and revert back to their previous eating ways.

Another reason why people quit a diet is because they become bored with their cooking because they can't include certain ingredients that used to make their food flavorful, and they feel that their options on what they can cook and eat are limited.

What makes the keto diet different to other diets is the fact that you are still able to eat most of the same types of foods that you could prior to starting the diet, with a few exceptions. You can easily substitute the foods that you should avoid, such as mashed potatoes, with those that you can eat, like cauliflower mash. Make sure to go back to the previous chapter and identify which foods you can swap out so that you are aware of all the possibilities as you cook.

I have collected 15 recipes in this chapter that you can use as a guide to getting started with cooking and eating healthy, tasty keto meals. These recipes will show you how to cook keto-friendly meals and how you can add flavor to keto dishes so that you never get bored.

Keto Quick and Easy Recipes

Starting the keto diet and learning how to cook food in new ways should not be hard, and the last thing you want to do after a long day is figure out what you want to cook and then spend hours cooking. Below, I have put together five quick and easy keto recipes that show you how simple cooking keto can be.

Keto Chicken, Broccoli, and Cauliflower Casserole

A keto broccoli and cauliflower casserole is a healthy low-carb keto meal that is easy to make and can quickly become your next guilty pleasure. This dish can be made for any occasion, whether you are entertaining or just cooking dinner, and can be served as a main meal or as a side.

If you do not like chicken, or if you just want a change, you can substitute the chicken in this casserole with an alternative meat option, such as bacon, ground beef, sausage, turkey, or vegan-friendly meat substitutes. Or you can enjoy this casserole without adding in any meat.

To store this casserole, you should first ensure that it has cooled down and then cover it and put it into the fridge to store for 3 to 4 days. It is not recommended that you store it in the freezer because the cream can become curdled when it defrosts.

Time: 40 minutes

Serving Size: ⅙ of casserole

Prep Time: 10 minutes

Cook Time: 30 minutes

Nutritional Facts/Info:

Calories 220

Carbs 9.8g

Fat 15.5g

Protein 12.2g

Ingredients:

- 1 medium head broccoli
- 1 medium head cauliflower
- ½ cup sour cream
- ¼ cup heavy cream

- 1 tsp Dijon mustard
- 1 tsp garlic powder
- ½ tsp salt, or to taste
- ¼ tsp black pepper, or to taste
- 1 rotisserie chicken, cooked and shredded
- 4 oz cheddar cheese, grated

Instructions:

1. Preheat the oven to 390°F.
2. Grease a casserole dish with olive oil.
3. On a cutting board, prepare the heads of broccoli and cauliflower by cutting out their stems and removing the leaves. Cut the broccoli and cauliflower into florets, place them in a colander, and wash them off in water.
4. Place water in a large pot and bring to the boil over high heat. Spoon the broccoli and cauliflower florets from the colander into the pot of water. Boil the florets until they are soft

enough that you can easily pierce them with a knife or fork.

5. While the broccoli and cauliflower florets are busy cooking, bring out a small saucepan and put it on the stove over low heat. Add in the sour cream, heavy cream, Dijon mustard, garlic powder, salt, and black pepper. Stir the ingredients together until they are well incorporated.

6. Once the broccoli and cauliflower are finished boiling, remove from the heat and drain the water from the pot. Switch the stove's plate to low heat and pour over the sauce that you have prepared in the saucepan and the shredded, cooked chicken.

7. Spoon the chicken, broccoli, and cauliflower mix into the casserole dish you prepared earlier and top with cheddar cheese.

8. Once the oven is preheated, place the dish inside and let it cook for 30 minutes until the cheese on top has turned a golden-brown color.
9. Take the casserole out of the oven and divide into six even pieces and serve.

Keto Lemon and Garlic Salmon with Green Beans

Eating foods that are high in healthy fats and oils is essential with the keto diet, and it is recommended that you include at least two meals in your diet per week that contain fatty fish to ensure you are meeting your recommended daily nutritional allowance. This lemon and garlic salmon with green beans tastes great, and it is quick and easy to make.

You can store leftovers in an airtight container or a Ziploc bag and keep it in the refrigerator for three to four days.

The recipe I have provided below can be made as a full meal on its own, or you can include other vegetables in this recipe as sides, such as vegetables like broccoli, cauliflower, spinach, or zucchini, or you can include a creamy cauliflower risotto. A broccoli and cheese bake would work well with this meal. I have included basic spices to season the salmon, but you can also use your own spices to make the salmon more to your tastes.

Time: 15 minutes

Serving Size: ¼ recipe

Prep Time: 5 minutes

Cook Time: 10 minutes

Nutritional Facts/Info:

Calories 617.7

Carbs 11.2g

Fat 42.4g

Protein 48.3g

Ingredients:

- 20 oz fresh green beans
- 6 oz butter
- 25 oz salmon cut into portions, or 4 salmon fillets
- 4 tsp garlic, crushed
- Salt to taste
- Black pepper to taste
- 1 lemon sliced

Instructions:

1. On a chopping board, cut off the ends of the green beans, place them into a colander, and wash them off. Put aside.
2. Put butter into a large frying pan on the stove over medium heat.
3. Put the fresh garlic into the butter and add in the green beans that you prepared and the salmon. Fry

the salmon on each side for 3 to 4 minutes, flipping the green beans a few times until the salmon has finished cooking. Spice the salmon with salt and black pepper to taste when you flip it over onto the next side.

4. When the salmon and green beans are finished cooking, remove the pan from the heat and serve on a plate with a slice of lemon.

Keto Burrito Lettuce Wrap

A low-carb keto burrito lettuce wrap is a great idea for a quick and easy lunch that you can take with you when you are on-the-go or that you and your family can have for dinner. Packed full of meat and bursting with flavor, everyone will love these burritos, even if they are not following the keto diet.

You can use beef strips, chicken, or ground beef for this recipe. If you want to, you can marinate the meat in an airtight container or a Ziploc bag in the fridge the evening before, or you can cook it as it is in a pan and serve, whichever is easiest for you. Along with the meat, you can add a selection of low-carb vegetables such as avocado, onions, bell peppers, and tomatoes, or any other vegetables that you like. Then you can top with some lemon juice, seeds, nuts, or any keto-friendly condiment before you roll the burrito closed.

I suggest that if you need to make these burritos the night before that you store the filling separately and take some lettuce leaves with you if you are on-the-go. If you make these up the night before, then the lettuce can become soggy by the time you want to eat it. You can heat up your filling before scooping it into the lettuce leaves and rolling it into a wrap. You can also eat your burrito as a burrito bowl or add it to a salad, if you are eating it the next day as leftovers.

Time: 20 minutes

Serving Size: 1 burrito

Prep Time: 10 minutes

Cook Time: 10 minutes

Nutritional Facts/Info:

Calories 436

Carbs 9.6g

Fat 32.9g

Protein 33g

Ingredients:

To make the meat marinade:

- ¼ cup olive oil
- 2 tbsp lemon juice, or lime juice
- 2 cloves garlic, crushed
- ½ tsp salt
- ¼ tsp cumin

128

- ¼ tsp oregano
- 1 lb beef steak strips or 1 lb chicken fillet strips

To make the burrito filling:

- 1 tbsp olive oil
- 1 onion, diced
- 2 cups peppers, sliced
- 1 tsp chili powder
- Salt to taste
- 18 leaves iceberg lettuce
- 1 avocado, diced
- ¾ cup shredded cheese

Instructions:

1. The night before or a few hours before you make your burritos, add olive oil, lemon juice or lime juice, garlic, salt, cumin, oregano, and meat to a Ziploc bag and seal it while pushing the air out. Then toss the meat around in the bag until it is well coated with the marinade. Set aside in the fridge.

2. The next day, or a few hours later, pour olive oil into a large frying pan on the stove over medium to high heat. Open the Ziploc bag with the meat that you previously marinated and pour into the pot. Add onions, peppers, and chili powder to the mixture. Taste the mixture and add more salt if there is not enough.

3. Fry the meat mixture on the stove until the meat browns and is fully cooked. This should take about 10 minutes. When the meat is finished cooking, remove from the heat and set aside.

4. You will need to use three large leaves of lettuce for each burrito that you are making. Take three lettuce leaves and lay them down, allowing them to overlap each other, on a cutting board or a plate.

5. Scoop the meat into the middle of the leaves of lettuce, leaving

space so that you can fold the bottom up. Try not to add too much meat to the lettuce, so that you do not overfill the burrito and can roll it closed. Add the avocado and cheese and see if anyone else wants any other fillings in their burrito.

6. Once everyone has decided on their filling, you can roll the burrito closed. Fold the bottom of the lettuce leaf upwards and then fold in one of the sides, and you can roll it the rest of the way until all the contents are tightly wrapped inside.

7. You can serve it as it is on a plate, or you can cut the burrito in half after wrapping it a second time in a sandwich paper to help hold it together if you are going to be handling the burrito without a plate, such as serving it when you are entertaining.

Keto Caprese Omelette

If you have some time in the mornings or over the weekend, you can make a quick keto caprese omelette. Not just for breakfast, this dish can also be served for lunch or even dinner. Like the classic caprese salad, this omelette comprises basil pesto, mozzarella cheese, and tomatoes covered in fresh balsamic vinegar.

If you are making this omelette for guests, you can serve this keto caprese omelette as the main meal with a salad or a fruit salad on the side. When serving this dish, you can add more basil pesto, mozzarella cheese, and tomatoes on top of the omelette.

Egg does not really refrigerate or freeze and then reheat nicely. I would suggest that you only make as much as you will be eating. This recipe will make two omelettes, so you should halve the recipe if you are only making one omelette for yourself.

Time: 10 minutes

Serving Size: 1 omelette

Prep Time: 5 minutes

Cook Time: 5 minutes

Nutritional Facts/Info:

Calories 457

Carbs 5.9g

Fat 35.9g

Protein 26.8g

Ingredients:

- 5 large eggs
- 1 cup cherry tomatoes, sliced into quarters
- 1 tbsp balsamic vinegar
- ½ tsp salt, or to taste
- ¼ tsp back pepper, or to taste

- ½ cup mozzarella cheese, grated
- ¼ cup basil pesto
- 2 tbsp parmesan cheese, grated

Instructions:

1. In a small mixing bowl, add the tomatoes, balsamic vinegar, salt, and pepper together and mix until well combined. Place the bowl aside.

2. In another small mixing bowl, crack open the eggs and whisk with a hand mixer or use a blender until the mixture is smooth and frothy. Place this bowl aside too.

3. Grease a large frying pan with olive oil or a keto-friendly nonstick cooking spray and put it on the stove over medium heat. Pour half of the egg mixture in the bowl you previously placed aside.

4. When you have added the egg mixture to the pan, let it cook for

about a minute, then add in half of the tomato and balsamic vinegar that you previously placed aside and top with mozzarella cheese.

5. Let the egg continue to cook until the egg is no longer runny and bubbles begin to form under the egg mixture's surface.

6. Lift an edge of the omelette away from the pan gently with a spatula and flip half of the omelette over onto the other side, covering it. Let the omelette cook for a further minute and then run the spatula under the other side of the omelette to separate it from the pan so that it does not stick.

7. Lift the omelette from the pan and place onto a plate. To serve, top the omelette with basil pesto, mozzarella cheese, a teaspoon of parmesan cheese, and tomatoes.

8. Repeat this process to create the second omelette.

Keto Bacon Cheeseburger Soup

For all of the flavor but with none of the carbs of an actual cheeseburger, this keto bacon cheeseburger soup is the ideal comfort food in winter and a perfect solution to indulge and fulfill your cravings without the guilt of cheating on your diet.

When serving the keto bacon cheeseburger soup, you can top the dish with bacon or leave it as it is as per your preference. If you choose to top the soup with bacon, you should bring out a pan and place it on the stove over high heat. Next, you will take 6 slices of bacon, dice them, and then add them into the pan. Then you will fry the bacon for 6 to 8 minutes until it has become crispy. Add the bacon on top of the soup and serve.

When storing your soup, you should wait for it to cool down and then transfer it from the pot to an airtight container. Soup should last 3 to 4 days in the refrigerator. To store in the freezer, you should choose a container that can handle the cold temperatures of the freezer or use a Ziploc bag. Soup should last 4 to 6 months in the freezer.

Time: 1 hour

Serving Size: ⅙ recipe

Prep Time: 15 minutes

Cook Time: 45 minutes

Nutritional Facts/Info:

Calories 365.4

Carbs 8g

Fat 32.4g

Protein 12.6g

Ingredients:

- 1 lb ground beef
- ½ onion, diced

- 2 garlic cloves, crushed
- 3 ½ cups beef broth
- 3 medium tomatoes
- 2 tbsp Worcestershire sauce
- 1 tbsp dried parsley
- 1 tsp dried dill
- 1 tsp mustard powder
- 1 tsp salt
- 4 oz cream cheese
- 1 ½ cups cheddar cheese, grated
- 1 cup heavy cream

Instructions:

1. Place olive oil in a pan and bring to medium heat over the stove. Add in the ground beef, onions, and garlic to the pan and fry them together until the ground beef browns and the onions become soft.
2. While the ground beef is cooking, dice an onion on a chopping board and set aside.
3. Once the ground beef is finished cooking, add in the beef broth,

diced tomatoes that you prepared, Worcestershire sauce, parsley, dill, mustard powder, and salt into the pan.

4. Stir the mixture of ingredients well and let the pan heat up and come to a boil before reducing the heat. Let it cook on low heat for 30 minutes.

5. After letting it cook for 30 minutes, add in the cream cheese and cheddar cheese, and pour in the heavy cream. Mix the ingredients together until the soup becomes creamy and thick.

6. Let the soup cool down before you serve it, and serve it as it is or add toppings of your choosing, such as bacon or additional cheddar cheese, onions, or tomatoes.

Tasty Keto Snacks and

Appetizers

When learning how to make keto food, it is a good idea to also learn some recipes to make some low-carb snacks as well. Whether you are making your own stash for when you have a craving for something to fill the gap before your next meal, or if you want to add a snack to your lunch bag, or even if you are making treats to serve to guests, these recipes are sure to be tasty and impress everyone who tries them.

Sour Lemon Gummies

Who does not love soft, chewy gummy sweets? They make the perfect snack when you are sitting down to watch a movie or just when you are craving a snack. These sour lemon gummies are bursting with flavor and will surely satisfy your taste buds.

You can also use this recipe to make other flavored gummy sweets, by replacing the lemon with strawberry, raspberry, blackberry, or blueberry. This recipe includes a sweetener, but you are welcome to not add in any; it all depends on what you prefer.

You can store these gummy sweets in an airtight container or a Ziploc bag. You can store them in a cool, dry place for up to two weeks. You do not need to store them in the refrigerator unless it gets quite humid where you live, and they stick to each other or if you prefer them cold. They also store for up to two weeks in the refrigerator.

Time: 1 hour 15 minutes

Serving Size: 10 gummy bears

Prep Time: 10 minutes

Cook Time: 5 minutes, with an hour to set

Nutritional Facts/Info:

Calories 9

Carbs 0.5g

Fat 0g

Protein 1.7g

Ingredients:

- 3 tbsp gelatin
- 2 tbsp powdered monkfruit
- ¼ cup fresh lemon juice
- ¼ cup water

Instructions:

1. Put a saucepan on the stove over low heat. Pour the water and lemon juice into the saucepan and add in the gelatin and monkfruit. Stir the mixture together until the gelatin

dissolves into the water and the mixture thickens into a paste.

2. Pour the mixture into a glass Pyrex measuring jug or a bowl with a spout that will not melt from the heat coming off the stove.

3. Pour the gummy mixture into silicone molds. In this recipe, we will be using a silicone gummy bear mold. But you can use any mold that you like. You should keep in mind that your number of servings and nutritional information will change depending on how big the shapes are in the mold and how many shapes are on each mold. You also do not have to use a mold. You can also pour the mixture out into a large Pyrex dish and cook it like that and cut it into similar strips.

4. Place the molds into the refrigerator and allow to cool for 1

hour. Once the gummies have set, you can push them out of their molds and store them.

Keto Jalapeño Poppers

Keto jalapeño poppers are a great snack that you can make for a barbeque or as a snack at a lunch or dinner gathering with friends and family. These keto jalapeño poppers pack a kick, are filled with cream cheese, and are topped with bacon. They taste delicious, are simple to make, and nobody would even guess they are keto-friendly.

You can make these keto jalapeño poppers ahead of time by preparing the jalapeños, cream cheese, and topping with bacon, then you can store them in the fridge. When your guests have arrived, or just before, you can pop them into the oven to start baking and serve piping hot.

If you have any leftovers, then you can store them in the fridge in an airtight container. You can reheat the jalapeño poppers by baking them a second time in the oven. They can also be stored in the freezer in a container that is safe to be placed in the freezer or a freezer bag, before you bake them, as well as after you bake them.

Time: 25 minutes

Serving Size: 1 jalapeño popper

Prep Time: 10 minutes

Cook Time: 15 minutes

Nutritional Facts/Info:

Calories 49

Carbs 1g

Fat 4g

Protein 2g

Ingredients:

- 6 medium jalapeños
- ¼ cup cheddar cheese, grated
- 3 oz cream cheese
- ¼ cup onions
- 2 cloves garlic
- 1 tsp olive oil
- 1 tbsp fresh cilantro
- ¼ cup bacon, diced

Instructions:

1. Preheat the oven to 400°F.
2. Roll out a silicone baking sheet, parchment paper, or foil onto a baking tray.
3. On a cutting board, slice the jalapeños lengthwise into two halves and place onto the baking tray.
4. Put olive oil into a frying pan on the stove over medium heat and add in the bacon. Allow the bacon to cook for a few minutes until browned.
5. While the bacon is busy cooking, take a small mixing bowl and add

in the cheddar cheese, cream cheese, onions, and garlic and mix together until it is well combined. If the bacon is finished cooking from earlier, remove it from the heat and put it aside.

6. Spoon the cheese mixture into each jalapeño half until all the halves have been filled. Top the jalapeño with the bacon you previously cooked and press it a bit into the jalapeño filling so that the pieces stick and do not fall off.

7. When the oven is finished preheating, put the jalapeños on the baking tray into the oven and let it bake for 15 minutes.

8. Once the jalapeño poppers are finished baking, take them out of the oven, place them on a plate, and serve.

Keto Egg Muffins

Keto egg muffins are healthy, versatile snacks that the whole family can enjoy. You can make them over the weekend to have for breakfast in the mornings if you are on-the-go, as quick, tasty snacks for you and your family when you are feeling peckish, or to keep your guests busy when you are entertaining.

There are many different fillings that you can use in your keto egg muffins, such as chicken and mushroom, broccoli and feta, and ham and cheese. I suggest that you use two or three variations of fillings when you make a batch so that you keep things interesting and get a new flavor whenever you pick one out.

These keto egg muffins are quick and easy to make. You can make them ahead of time, such as over the weekend to eat throughout the week, or the night before an event.

148

Once you have taken the keto egg muffins out of the oven, you should let them stand and cool before placing them into a Ziploc plastic bag or an airtight container. They can keep for five days in the fridge, and three months in the freezer.

Time: 25 minutes

Serving Size: 1 muffin

Prep Time: 10 minutes

Cook Time: 15 minutes

Nutritional Facts/Info:

Calories 100.3

Carbs 0.9g

Fat 7g

Protein 7.9g

Ingredients:

- 10 large eggs

- 1 tsp salt
- 1/2 tsp black pepper
- 1/2 tsp onion powder (optional)
- 1/2 tsp garlic powder (optional)
- 1/3 cup onion, chopped
- 2/3 cup cheddar cheese, grated
- 2/3 cup ham, diced

Instructions:

1. Preheat the oven to 400°F.
2. Take out a muffin tray with space for 12 muffins and spray it with nonstick spray or line it with silicon or paper cups. Set aside.
3. Break the eggs open into a medium-sized mixing bowl and add salt and pepper. Using a hand blender or whisk, beat the mixture until it is well combined.
4. To add a different taste to the egg muffins, you can season the egg mixture with onion and garlic powder. This step is optional and can be skipped.

5. Divide and spoon onions, cheddar cheese, and ham into the muffin cups. Do not put too much filling into the muffin cups but rather aim to fill each halfway.
6. Pour the egg mixture into each of the muffin cups until each is 2/3 full.
7. When the preheated oven is ready, place the muffin tray into the oven and cook for 12 to 15 minutes until firm.
8. Remove the muffin tray from the oven and let it cool for five minutes. If you are not using silicon or paper cups, then you can use a knife and slide it around each cup so that the muffins do not stick when you take them out of the cups.

Bacon-Wrapped Halloumi Cheese

These bacon-wrapped halloumi cheese fingers are a great addition to any gathering. They are keto-friendly, quick and easy to make, and are well-loved by both those following a keto diet and those who are nonketo. These bacon-wrapped halloumi cheese fingers also make an excellent midnight snack, minus the guilt that comes with it! Be sure to save yourself some for the next day when you make them as a snack.

If you do not want to bake them or if you want a change, you can also fry these in a pan with some olive oil or butter over medium-to-high heat. You can serve this as a side to a bigger meal or as finger food with a dip to add more flavor and depth to it. You can substitute bacon in this dish with pancetta. You can top the dish off by adding a splash of lemon juice.

To store, you should wait for them to cool down and then put them into an airtight container or Ziploc bag without any toppings. You can store these in the fridge for up to two to three days and a bit longer in the freezer. The halloumi and bacon should stay together well when reheating, but you can stick a toothpick through it if you are worried that it will come apart.

Time: 25 minutes

Serving Size: 1 cheese finger

Prep Time: 10 minutes

Cook Time: 15 minutes

Nutritional Facts/Info:

Calories 89

Carbs 1g

Fat 5g

Protein 4g

Ingredients:

- 25 oz halloumi cheese
- 20 oz bacon, in strips or sliced

Instructions:

1. Preheat the oven to 400°F.
2. Line an oven tray with a silicone mat or parchment paper and set aside.
3. Place the halloumi cheese on a chopping board and cut it lengthwise into 12 thin, even strips. Gather the halloumi in a corner on the chopping board so that there is more space for you to work.
4. Take a strip of bacon and lay it out flat on the chopping board. If your pack of bacon has wide cuts of bacon that are as big as your halloumi cheese fingers, then you should cut them lengthwise to halve them before you continue. Once you have enough bacon, you

can place a finger of halloumi cheese on top of the bacon and wrap the bacon along the length of the halloumi cheese finger.

5. Place the bacon-wrapped halloumi cheese fingers onto the prepared oven tray.

6. Once the oven has been preheated, place the tray into the oven and let it cook for 7 minutes, and then take it out and turn them before returning the tray to the oven to cook for another 7 minutes until fully cooked and crispy.

7. When they are finished cooking, remove from the oven and serve.

Keto Cheddar Cheese and Bacon Balls

These tasty keto cheddar cheese and bacon balls make for the perfect appetizers to wow your guests. They are low carb and packed with healthy fats and protein. These balls work best when served chilled or at room temperature.

You can substitute the cheddar cheese in these balls with any other cheese options, such as colby jack, gouda, monterey jack, mozzarella, and swiss. For a bit of a bite, you can add some finely grated or diced jalapeños to your cheese mix. If you or any of your friends are vegetarian or vegan, then you can roll these cheese balls in crushed nuts or seeds instead of bacon.

You can serve these balls with some toothpicks so that your guests can get themselves a serving more easily, and a pot of spices on the side to change the taste and texture of the balls, such as a seasoning, or a pot of keto-friendly homemade sauce that they can dip their balls into.

These keto cheddar cheese and bacon balls can be stored in an airtight container or Ziploc bag in the fridge for three to four days and can easily be stored in the freezer in a freezer-safe container or freezer bag for longer. When you want to eat them again, you should let them warm to room temperature.

Time: 20 minutes

Serving Size: 1 keto cheddar cheese and bacon ball

Prep Time: 15 minutes

Cook Time: 5 minutes

Nutritional Facts/Info:

Calories 274

Carbs 2g

Fat 26g

Protein 8g

Ingredients:

- 5 oz bacon, finely diced
- 1 tbsp butter
- 5 oz cream cheese
- 5 oz cheddar cheese, grated
- 2 oz butter
- ½ tsp pepper
- ½ tsp chili flakes

Instructions:

1. Put butter into a frying pan on the stove over medium heat and add the bacon to the pan. Fry the bacon until fully cooked and crispy. Once cooked, remove from the heat and scoop the bacon out into a separate bowl.
2. In a large mixing bowl, add the bacon grease from the pan, as well as the cream cheese, cheddar

cheese, pepper, and chili flakes. Mix these ingredients by hand until they are well combined. If you do not want to use your hands, you can use an electric hand mixer or a standing mixer.

3. Once the ingredients have been mixed thoroughly, put the mixing bowl into the fridge to chill for 15 minutes.

4. After 15 minutes, remove the mixing bowl from the fridge and use two spoons to scoop out 24 balls that are about the size of a walnut. You can reshape the balls with your hands if they come out unevenly. Once you have formed your cheddar cheese and bacon balls, roll them into the bowl with the cooked bacon in to coat them.

5. Serve to your guests or enjoy as a snack.

Keto   Meals   for

Entertaining

Entertaining guests and cooking food for people can be tricky, and that was already before you started the keto diet. I have compiled a few recipes below that you can use to create delicious low-carb, keto-friendly dishes that will amaze your friends. With these recipes, your friends and family will be asking you to host gatherings just so that they can eat your yummy keto dishes!

Keto Cauliflower Potato Salad

Having a classic potato salad at a gathering or a barbeque is a must. But what happens when you cannot eat potatoes? You can make a quick, low-carb keto-friendly cauliflower "potato" salad instead, of course. This keto cauliflower potato salad is the perfect salad for any occasion. At first thought, you might not think that this dish would go well together, but it tastes great and your guests are sure to think so too!

You can top this dish with some chopped green onions, chives, and a keto-friendly seasoning spice to give it a bite of flavor. Some meat toppings that you might like to add to this dish include bacon, tuna, or some shredded chicken meat.

You can store this salad in an airtight container in the fridge for three to four days and help yourself to servings when you want them. I do not suggest that you store it in the freezer, as the mayonnaise in the cauliflower salad will not thaw in an appetizing way.

Time: 15 minutes

Serving Size: ⅕ recipe

Prep Time: 5 minutes

Cook Time: 10 minutes

Nutritional Facts/Info:

Calories 250

Carbs 11g

Fat 21g

Protein 6g

Ingredients:

- 1 large head cauliflower
- ⅔ cup mayonnaise
- 1 tbsp apple cider vinegar
- 1 tbsp Dijon mustard
- ½ tsp garlic powder
- ½ tsp paprika
- ½ tsp salt, or to taste

- ¼ tsp black pepper, or to taste
- ⅓ cup onion, finely diced
- ⅓ cup celery, finely diced
- 2 large egg, hard boiled, chopped

Instructions:

1. On a chopping board, prepare the cauliflower by cutting out the stem and removing the leaves, and discard them both.
2. Chop the cauliflower into florets, place into a colander, and wash them off with water. Set aside.
3. Put water into a large pot and place on the stove over medium heat. Add a dash of salt to the pot of water and bring to a boil. When the water is bubbling, add in the cauliflower florets that you prepared earlier and cook for 5 minutes until soft. You can poke at a floret with a fork or a knife to check how soft it has become.
4. While the cauliflower is busy cooking, take out a large bowl and

add the mayonnaise, apple cider vinegar, Dijon mustard, garlic powder, paprika, salt, and black pepper. Stir the mixture together until the texture is smooth and well combined and set aside.

5. Once the cauliflower is finished cooking, remove from the heat and drain the water.

6. Pour the cauliflower into the bowl and combine the cauliflower florets into the mayonnaise mixture. Add in the onion, celery, and egg and give it another good stir to make sure that all the ingredients are evenly distributed in the salad.

7. You can garnish with paprika and chives, and add any toppings that you would like, and then serve.

Keto Shrimp and Cauliflower Risotto

Eating shrimp is a great way to include healthy omega-3 fats and oils into your diet. Paired with a lemon butter sauce, this keto shrimp and cauliflower risotto is comforting and delicious. Whether you are cooking for the family or entertaining, this creamy low-carb dish is sure to be a crowd pleaser.

You can serve this dish on its own with slices or wedges of lemon for yourself or your guests to add extra lemon to their fish and risotto. You can garnish the meal with bacon, or you can add chives. If you do not want shrimp in this dish, you can substitute the shrimp with cod, haddock, hake, mackerel, salmon, and trout, or whichever fish you think would go well with this.

To store, let the food cool down first and then place it into an airtight container. You can keep this meal in your fridge for three to four days before it goes bad and you have to throw it out. Do not take chances with seafood if it has been longer than three or four days, as you can get food poisoning.

Time: 30 minutes

Serving Size: ¼ recipe

Prep Time: 10 minutes

Cook Time: 20 minutes

Nutritional Facts/Info:

Calories 397.1

Carbs 17.4 g

Fat 28.8 g

Protein 20.7 g

Ingredients:

- 3 tbsp olive oil
- 1 onion, diced
- 1 1/2 tsp salt

- 1/2 tsp black pepper
- 1 tsp dried thyme
- 2 cloves of garlic, crushed
- 2 cups vegetable stock
- 1 large head cauliflower
- 3 tbsp butter
- 1 tbsp lemon juice
- 8 oz shrimp
- ¼ cup heavy cream
- ½ cup parmesan cheese, grated

Instructions:

1. Place olive oil in a pan and bring to medium heat on the stove. Add the onions, salt, black pepper, and dried thyme into the pan and let it cook until the onions start to brown and become soft.

2. While the onions are busy cooking, you can prepare the head of cauliflower by cutting out the stem and removing the leaves. Cut the cauliflower into florets, place them into a colander, and wash them off with water.

3. Divide the cauliflower florets into batches and blitz each batch in a food processor until they are about the size of rice grains. Put aside.

4. Add garlic in with the onions that have been cooking on the stove and allow the flavor to infuse with the other ingredients in the pan for 1 to 2 minutes.

5. Add the cauliflower that you previously prepared with the onion and garlic mixture in the pan and mix it together until it is evenly combined.

6. Pour vegetable stock into the pan and let it simmer for 5 minutes with the lid on, and then an additional 5 to 10 minutes with the lid removed until excess liquid has cooked down.

7. Grease another pan with butter, add in the shrimp, and cook for 2 to 4 minutes or until they start to turn a lighter pink color.

8. Add the lemon juice, ⌐
   parmesan cheese to the
   stir until it forms a crear.
9. Serve your dish onto a ⸝
   let your guests add th ⸝wn
   toppings, or any garnishing or
   condiments they would like.
   Enjoy!
10. Alternatively, you can serve your
    meal on a plate and let your
    guests add their own toppings.

Keto Indian Chicken Curry

You will definitely be turning some
heads when you make this hearty keto
Indian chicken curry. This low-carb
chicken curry is mild, easy to make, full
of many healthy fats, and is bursting
with flavor. This dish works well for
both a lunch or dinner gathering, or as a
warming winter meal for yourself and
your family.

This recipe is for a chicken curry, but the chicken can be replaced by another meat, such as beef cubes, fish, or lamb. For your vegetarian friends, you can replace the meat in this dish with tofu. You can serve this dish with a side, such as keto cauliflower rice, or some other nonstarchy vegetables. You can add in more chilis when you are cooking this dish to give it more of a bite, if you want a hotter curry.

If you have any leftovers, you should wait for it to cool down, then place it in an airtight container and store it in the fridge for one week. If you want to freeze your leftovers, you should place them into a freezer-safe container or a freezer bag, and store for three months. When you want to warm leftovers from the freezer, you should transfer it to the fridge and let it thaw, then you can warm it up and serve it.

Time: 55 minutes

Serving Size: ⅛ recipe

Prep Time: 15 minutes

Cook Time: 40 minutes

Nutritional Facts/Info:

Calories 414

Carbs 4g

Fat 36g

Protein 20g

Ingredients:

- 1 small onion, diced
- 1 green chili, chopped
- 3 cloves garlic
- 1-inch knob of ginger, chopped
- ½ cup fresh coriander, with leaves and stems
- 3 tbsp of ghee, or butter
- 2 tsp turmeric, ground
- 1 ½ tsp cumin, ground
- 1 tsp coriander, ground
- 2 tbsp tomato paste

- 2 lb chicken breasts, diced
- 1 cup heavy cream
- 1 tsp salt, or to taste

Instructions:

1. Take a medium-sized mixing bowl, and add in the onion, green chili, garlic, ginger, and coriander. Using a hand blender, blitz these ingredients together until they have been processed more finely. If you have a food processor, then you can add these ingredients into the food processor and do the same. You can add a splash of water to help you process the ingredients. Place aside.

2. Put the ghee into a large saucepan on the stove over low heat. Scoop the mixture out of the mixing bowl or processor and combine it with the ghee. Allow the onion and chili mix to cook in

the ghee for 10 minutes, stirring often.

3. Add turmeric, cumin, and coriander to the onion and chili ingredients in the pan and continue to stir it in and cook in the ghee for an additional 5 minutes.

4. Add in the tomato paste and mix with the ingredients until well combined. Continue to stir and cook the mixture for 2 more minutes, then add in the chicken.

5. When you add the chicken to the ingredients in the pan, turn the stove up to medium heat and allow the chicken to cook and be coated by the spices for 10 minutes.

6. After 10 minutes, reduce the stove's heat and add the cream and salt into the saucepan. Allow the chicken to continue to simmer on low heat for 20 to 25 minutes, letting the sauce

Jnce the chicken is fully
remove from the heat.
.ve, dish up your chicken
/ into a bowl and serve with a
e dish, such as cauliflower rice.

Keto Beef Tacos

Get ready to entertain and make a bang
with a Mexican taco night and make
keto beef tacos that taste so great that
your guests will not even believe it is
keto. These beef tacos are low carb and
keto friendly, not to mention easy to
make.

You can serve the keto beef tortillas with
avocado, cheddar cheese, parmesan
cheese, lettuce, and tomatoes. You can
also top the tortillas off with keto-
friendly condiments.

When storing tacos, you can put them
into an airtight container and put them

into the fridge. They can last for 3 to 4 days in the fridge. When reheating your taco shell, it might not have the same crunchy texture that it had when you first made the tacos.

Time: 50 minutes

Serving Size: ¼ recipe

Prep Time: 20 minutes

Cook Time: 20 - 30 minutes

Nutritional Facts/Info:

Calories 432

Carbs 7g

Fat 33g

Protein 28g

Ingredients:

- 9 oz cheddar cheese, grated
- 1 lb ground beef
- 1 tbsp chile powder

- 1 ½ tsp cumin
- 1 tsp paprika
- ½ tsp garlic powder
- ½ tsp dried onion
- ½ tsp oregano
- 1 tsp salt, or to taste
- ½ tsp black pepper, or to taste
- 2 tbsp tomato paste
- ½ cup beef broth

Instructions:

1. Preheat the oven to 350°F.
2. Prepare 2 large sheet pans with silicone mats or parchment paper.
3. Spoon the cheddar cheese in three similarly shaped circles on the silicone mats or parchment paper. They do not have to be perfect, and they should be about 6 inches each in size. If you struggle to get the shape right, you can draw out the three circles on the back of the parchment paper to help guide you.

4. Once the oven has been preheated, you can bake the cheese circles for 6 to 8 minutes until they turn golden brown. I suggest that you put the sheet pans in one at a time, but you do not have to.

5. While the cheese circles are busy baking, grease a pan with olive oil and put it on the stove over medium temperature. Add the ground beef into the pan and break it apart, browning it. Once the ground beef has cooked, add in your spices, chile powder, cumin, paprika, garlic powder, dried onion, oregano, salt, and pepper. Stir the ground beef mix to spread the spices throughout the meat. Add tomato paste and beef broth into the pan and mix until well combined and the sauce thickens.

6. When you have finished cooking the ground beef filling, you can

remove it from the heat and put it aside.

7. Once the cheese circles are finished baking, you should let them cool down for a minute or two, and then place them into a taco shaper to help bend the cheese circle into a taco shape. You should let them cool in the taco shaper for 10 minutes before removing them. Remove the cheese shells and replace them until all of them have been shaped. If you do not have a taco shaper, you can use two glasses or other sturdy raised objects and a wooden spoon and balance the spoon between the glasses. You will then need to place the cheese circle over the wooden spoon to shape it into the right shape.

8. To serve, spoon the ground beef filling into the cheese shells and serve. Allow your guests to add

their own garnishes
as they prefer.

Keto Frittata with Fresh Spinach

A frittata is made to be shared, whether you are cooking lunch for your family, or if you are having an intimate teatime gathering at your house with your friends. This keto frittata with fresh spinach is low carb and easy to make. Packed with nutrients, this frittata has bacon, eggs, spinach, and vegetables. It is a light meal that you can have for breakfast or lunch and is gentle on your stomach, while leaving you feeling satiated.

You can substitute the bacon in this recipe with sausage like chorizo, or you can add both bacon and chorizo to the frittata to change things up. If you do not feel like making a large frittata, or if you are looking to have one in the mornings or for lunch when you are on-the-go, you can make these on a smaller scale in muffin tins. You can serve your frittata as it is, or you could serve with a keto-friendly condiment that goes well with the frittata.

Once your frittata has cooled down, you can store it in an airtight container in your fridge for three to four days. When storing it in your freezer, you can store it in a container that is freezer-safe or in a freezer bag, if you have one that is large enough, or you can divide the frittata into portions. When you want to serve your frittata, you should let it thaw in the fridge for 24 hours before serving it.

Time: 45 minutes

Serving Size: ¼ recipe

Prep Time: 10 minutes

Cook Time: 35 minutes

Nutritional Facts/Info:

Calories 661

Carbs 4g

Fat 59g

Protein 27g

Ingredients:

- 5 oz bacon, diced
- 2 tbsp butter
- 8 oz fresh spinach
- 8 eggs
- 1 cup heavy cream
- 5 oz cheddar cheese, grated
- ½ tsp salt, or to taste
- ¼ tsp black pepper, or to taste

Instructions:

1. Preheat the oven to 350°F.
2. Grease a round baking dish with olive oil or a keto-friendly nonstick cooking spray.
3. Put butter into a frying pan on the stove over medium heat. Add

in the bacon and fry until it is cooked and has become crispy.

4. Add the spinach into the pan with the bacon and mix until the spinach becomes to droop and get soggy. Once the bacon and spinach are finished cooking, remove from the heat and place it aside.

5. In a mixing bowl, break open the eggs, add the cream, and beat until it forms a smooth, golden consistency.

6. Pour the egg and cream mixture into the round baking dish and top with the bacon and spinach that was previously set aside. Also top with cheese.

7. Once the oven has been preheated, place the baking dish inside the oven and bake for 25 to 30 minutes until the egg has set and it becomes a golden-brown color. You can use a sharp knife to check if the frittata has cooked

through completely. To do this, push the tip of the knife into the center of the frittata. If the knife comes back clear, then it is finished cooking. If not, you will need to cook it for the additional 5 minutes and then check again.

8. When it is finished cooking, remove from the oven and allow it to cool down. Then cut the frittata into four slices and serve.

Chapter 6: Maintaining Your Keto Lifestyle

When there is so much going on in your life, it might become difficult to stick to a diet. However, you should approach the keto diet with the mindset that you are making a lifestyle change, and not that you are looking for a quick fix by following the rules of a diet. When you change your mindset and begin to incorporate the diet into various aspects of your life, you will truly begin to appreciate what you are working towards and the health benefits that you can experience by maintaining your keto lifestyle.

Dining Out

184

Being on a keto diet does not mean that you can now never eat out again or go out with your friends and enjoy yourself. You should be able to have fun, enjoy good food, and do all of the things that you love to do, otherwise your diet will feel like a prison, and you will find yourself eating cheat meals more often and going back and forth between the keto diet and not seeing any changes. Below are a few tips that you can use to eat out with the keto diet.

Plan Ahead

Before you head out or order in, you should take a look and see if there are any keto restaurants or restaurants that offer keto-friendly food options that are near your location. You can check this using Google or Yelp, or by typing in the keyword "keto" when searching for food on any food ordering app. Restaurants that should have keto-friendly foods are burger restaurants, Mexican restaurants, places that sell breakfast and brunch options, and places that have salad bars.

You should also make sure that you take a look at each restaurant's menu to check if there are any meals or other food items that are either marked keto or sound like they could be keto friendly. Many restaurants have updated their menus to include this type of information to help their customers who have specific dietary requirements order food. You can also call the restaurant if you are unsure about anything or if you have any questions before you place your order online or go out.

Ordering

If you do not have much of a choice and you are ordering in or eating out at a nonketo restaurant, then you will need to select your meals carefully when you are placing your order. You should take some time and go through each item on their menu if you were not able to do so before online.

When ordering nonketo foods, you should look at the food options that have little to no carbs included in the dish, or carbs that can be removed from the dish. You should choose a meal that includes some nonstarchy vegetables like arugula, asparagus, bell peppers, broccoli, brussels sprouts, cauliflower, kale, mushrooms, spinach, and tomatoes, healthy fats like avocado, and a moderate amount of protein.

When checking through their menu, you should also be aware that there are some foods that are prepared in such a way that they include added sugar and carbohydrates while they are cooking the food. Some examples of how restaurants can include added sugar and carbohydrates into a dish include coating some foods with a non-keto-friendly breading, using croutons in salads, adding syrup or jam to dishes to give them a sweet flavor, using tomato sauce or paste to give some foods an extra tangy tomato taste, thickening sauces with flour, pouring gravy over a dish, serving a dish with dried fruit, and using potatoes in some dishes, like soup and stew.

If you remove starch from a meal, such as asking them to not include a potato bake in a meal, and you are now only left with protein and nonstarchy vegetables on your plate, you should consider adding a side that is high in fat, such as avocado or egg. You could also ask them to add some butter or olive oil that can go over your vegetables, if they do not have many sides that they can offer you that are high in fats.

Another thing you should check for before you order is for condiments and other sauces. Condiments and other sauces can have many added sugars contained in them. If possible, you can ask them what they made the sauce with, or if they can remove the sauce or put it separately and not mixed in or drizzled over the food. If you order steak, you should make sure that they do not cook it with a basting like BBQ sauce and ask them to season it using only salt, pepper, and whichever other keto-friendly spice that you like that they do not mind doing for you. Otherwise, you can ask them to cook it without any spices or sauces and add your own when it arrives at your table.

There are many beverages that you should avoid on the keto diet. One can never be sure what a restaurant or takeaway puts into their drinks, so you should try to avoid drinking most of their beverage options. Beverages that you can include when ordering are infused water with cucumber, lemon, or lime, soda water, sparkling water, water, and unsweetened tea and coffee. You should ensure that they do not give you milk with your tea or coffee or ask them if they can bring you some heavy cream instead. You can add sweetener to your tea and coffee, to your taste.

If you cannot find any meals on their menu to your tastes or which are not keto friendly, then you can order a few of their sides, such as a side salad, cooked vegetables, olives, a boiled egg, scrambled egg, bacon, an omelette, sausage, and so on. If you mix a few of the different sides that they offer together, you can make your own keto-friendly meal.

If you are ever unsure about what is in a specific meal or how the restaurant prepares certain foods, then you can always ask. Most restaurant employees are happy to give you a rundown of their foods, and sometimes if they are not too busy, they can prepare a more keto-friendly version of one of their meals for you. So, do not be afraid to ask them questions.

There are some wonderful keto-friendly dessert recipes out there. However, when you go to a nonketo restaurant, you will need to look for other alternatives, especially if your group wants to stay for dessert, or you are craving something sweet when ordering from home. You should try to avoid the restaurant's dessert menu and check if they have some other options. You may need to ask someone at the restaurant if they would mix some things together for you, but you can look through the menu as well. Some dessert ideas you could order include herbal tea, a cheese platter, dark chocolate, some berries served in cream, or a decaf coffee with cream.

When I go out, I like to order a rump or sirloin steak with a side green salad or a side of cooked vegetables, such as spinach or any other nonstarchy vegetable. If you order a side salad, then you should check to make sure you can eat all the vegetables that are included in the salad, especially if you have removed a few food items from the salad. Not all salads are the same depending on the restaurant you order from, but you can generally eat a green salad without worrying if it is keto friendly. Also, if you order a cooked vegetable side, you should ask how it is prepared to make sure that they do not include any added sugars or carbohydrates in the cooking process.

Just in Case

When you have been doing the keto diet for a while, you will become more familiar with the restaurants in your area and whether they have any keto-friendly options or not. If you know that you might struggle to find something at a restaurant when you are meeting up with your friends, then you might need to eat something before you leave the house and then order a side that you can nibble on while your friends are eating. That way, you will not feel left out by your friends, nor will you be hungry.

In less formal situations, such as going for a picnic or hike with friends and family, or visiting your family for a Sunday lunch, you can prepare your own meals to take with you if they are fine with you doing this (which they should not have a problem with). By doing this, you do not need to rely on anyone preparing you a separate lunch that is keto-friendly when everyone else is eating something else.

Breaking a Weight Loss Plateau

Everyone reaches a weight loss plateau at some point in their diet, where they no longer see any more progress towards their health and weight loss goals. If you notice that you are experiencing a weight loss plateau, then you should think about what could be causing it. Maybe you are working out and losing weight, but replacing that weight with muscle mass. Or perhaps you are losing inches around your waist, arms, and hips, and you are not noticing it because you cannot see the weight loss on the scale.

Here are a few tips and tricks that you can use to break a weight loss plateau and continue seeing weight loss as you follow the keto diet:

- **Keep track of the carbs you eat each day.** To get your body into ketosis, you should be including 20 grams of carbohydrates in your diet each day. However, if you are not in ketosis, you can have up to 50 grams of carbohydrates each day. You should use a food and calorie tracking app to keep track of how many calories and carbohydrates you are eating each day. A food and calorie tracking app can let you know if you are eating too many carbohydrates each day, and you can see which foods are high in carbohydrates and cut them out or replace them in your diet.

- **Take a break from restricting your carbohydrates.** Sometimes you are not losing weight because you are trying too hard to lose weight. If you are constantly in ketosis and restricting your carbohydrate intake to 20 grams or less each day, you might risk slowing down your metabolism and hitting a weight loss plateau. If this happens to you, you should take a break from restricting your carbohydrates for a week or two to help kick-start your ketosis and fat burning and get your metabolism going again.

- **Celebrate the small victories.** If you have been doing everything right, and the numbers on the scale have not budged, and you have not noticed any more weight loss, then you might not be looking at your weight loss in the right way. The next time you do a weigh-in, take your measurements with a tape measure and then take them again the next time. You might notice that you have lost a few inches around your waist, hips, arms, and so on, and you would not have noticed this by just checking the figures on the scale. When you notice you have lost some inches in a few places, you should continue to be positive and stick to it and not be discouraged. It will all be worth it in the end!

- **Decrease your calorie deficit.** If you are not already using a food and calorie tracking app, I really recommend it. You can set your calorie intake to your own specific goals. You should work out how many calories you need each day and add in all the foods you eat throughout the day. This kind of application can easily tell you if you have a calorie deficit in your diet each day, which may be the reason why you are not losing any more weight. You should try and cut a few things out of your diet to decrease your calorie deficit or spend more time exercising to burn these extra calories off.
- **Eat the right amount of protein.** You should not eat too much or too little protein in your

diet. When you eat too little protein, you can lose muscle mass, experience cravings, and feel hungry more often, and you will not have as much energy, which can cause your weight loss to decrease. If you eat too much protein, you will not release as many ketones, and your body will switch to rely more on sugar to provide your body with energy, causing you to have sugar cravings. Making sure that you eat the right amount of protein each day is important for weight loss and to ensure that you do not hit a weight loss plateau.

- **Stay consistent.** By sticking to your diet and staying consistent, you will increase the rate at which you lose weight and keep your body in a ketosis cycle. If you are inconsistent and constantly cycling into and out of ketosis and if you have cheat meals, it can take your body time to recover and get back to creating and burning ketones in your body. You should be mindful of this as you start your keto diet and realize that if you are having cheat days or your diet is not consistent, then you will not lose as much weight and can hit a weight loss plateau quickly into your diet.

- **Start exercising and being more active.** There is a chance that you might have hit a weight loss plateau because you are inactive. Weight loss is 80% of what you put into your body and 20% exercise and getting active. If you are struggling to lose stubborn weight, you should organize a workout schedule to get you moving and exercising. To see the best results with the keto diet, you should do weight training at least twice a week, with 30-minute aerobic workouts, such as cycling, running, swimming, and walking for the days you are not doing weight training. You should ensure that you include one or two days to rest as well, so that your body can recover.

- **Try intermittent fasting.** As we go about our day, we eat our main meals and then eat a few snacks in between. These snacks might be small, and because they are keto, you think that it is fine to have them in your diet and that you will not pick up weight. But these extra carbohydrates and fats can sneak up on you and might be the reason why you are not losing weight. To get back onto the weight loss wagon, you should cut these snacks out of your diet and focus on eating only your main meals, which are breakfast, lunch, and dinner. You should also make sure that you time when you eat certain foods. If you have a meal with carbs in it for dinner and then are not active for the rest of the evening and go to bed, then those carbs have no way of being burned by your body as energy and will be converted into stored fat. Instead, you should rather move your carbohydrates into your breakfast or lunch meals, and try not to have any in the evening. That way, the carbohydrates that you eat will have a chance to be burned off throughout the day as energy. Another way that you can lose weight in this way is by doing intermittent fasting by eating within a certain time period, for example between 11am and 7pm, and then you do not eat anything before then, or after then. During this time, you will space out two or three meals. So, for example, you will have breakfast, a snack, and then lunch with no second snack or dinner. You can also switch it around and have your lunch, a snack, and then dinner with no breakfast. By eating in this way, you can teach your body to burn more fat, and you will notice that you do not feel as hungry or have as many cravings as before.

- **Try fat fasting.** Another type of fasting that you can try is a fat fast, where you eat between 1,000 to 1,200 calories each day for two to four days, with 80 to 90% of the calories that you consume coming from fats. Fat fasting can kick-start your metabolism and increase the amount of ketones that your body produces.

- **Look for hidden carbs.** Foods that might say that they are low carb or keto friendly could still have hidden carbs in them. Make sure that you check the nutritional information for all the food that you buy to make sure that there are no added sugars or carbohydrates. You should check that if foods have carbohydrates in them that they are under 5 grams of net carbs per food item and that starch and sugar are not listed in the first five ingredients on the ingredients list. Take a look at chapter five for more information on reading nutritional information and labels. If a food item has too many carbs, you should try and substitute it with a similar product that has less carbs in it.

- **Avoid sweeteners and low-carb treats.** Another reason why you may not be losing weight could be because you are including too many sweeteners and low-carb snacks and treats in your diet. Something that you should always remember, especially when you buy things from shops that claim that something is "low carb" or "keto friendly," is that this does not mean that it does not contain any sweeteners or that the carbohydrate intake is under 5 grams. Unless you are baking yourself and checking each recipe, then that sweet keto treat you got from the shop might be the reason you are not losing weight. Try to avoid buying sweet treats, or try not to eat them too often. Also, if you are having more than one cup of coffee a day, you should cut the sweetener from your coffee. Sweeteners still contain sugar, and although the sugar content is very low, it can all add up if you have three cups of coffee a day with two or more sweeteners in them each time.

- **Stress and sleepless nights.** Unrelated to food, your weight loss could have plateaued due to stress and not getting enough sleep. When this happens, the cortisol in your body increases, which also increases your cravings for high-carb foods and makes you feel hungry more often. This can cause you to gain weight. If you are stressed, there are a few methods that you can use to reduce your stress, such as exercise, breathing exercises, playing relaxing music before bed, and so on. If you are still battling with stress and insomnia, you should see your general practitioner to see what can be done to alleviate your stress and help you sleep better at night.

Conclusion

Following a keto diet is not simply a quick fix, and it is highly suggested that you follow it with the intention of making it a lifelong lifestyle change. The keto diet is healthy for you and has the ability to assist your body through the changes that you will be experiencing as you turn 50 and older. Because you are not just cutting out carbohydrates completely from your diet, your body will still be receiving all the nutrients that it needs to sustain you.

The keto diet has become very popular, for younger and older people alike, so you should not have many problems finding a keto community or group that can give you the advice that you need, answer your questions, and even meet up from time to time to share their experiences and well-loved keto recipes.

To find more support on the keto diet, you should join a few groups on Facebook to meet like-minded people who share your lifestyle goals and ideals. You can also look for new recipes online and in cookbooks. I like to buy a new cookbook every once in a while and play a game. I will take the cookbook, close my eyes, and flip through the pages. Whichever page my finger lands on, I will try that recipe and see how it is and make a note of what recipe I tried so that it is easy to come back to later.

You would be surprised to find out how many blogs there are that are dedicated to creating and writing about keto-friendly recipes. What I love about these blogs is that they often provide you with a printable recipe at the end of the blog page that details all the information about the recipe, including nutritional information. You can print out your favorite recipes like this and add them to a file to refer back to later.

If you are faced with any difficult situations when following the keto diet, you should remind yourself of why you started the keto diet to begin with and what you are hoping to see from your diet health-wise or lifestyle-wise. No matter what your reason is for starting the keto diet, you should focus on that and try to put difficult situations behind you. If you are still having trouble coping with a certain situation, then you can always ask for advice from one of your keto groups or your like-minded friends. You never know, they might have some great advice for you.

Do Not Go Yet; One Last Thing to Do
If you enjoyed this book or found it useful,
I'd be very grateful if you'd post a short
review on Amazon. Your support does make
a difference, and I read all the reviews
personally so I can get your feedback and
make this book even better.

Thanks again for your support!

Printed in Great Britain
by Amazon

45888965R00119